J. DAUGAARD

SYMPTOMS AND SIGNS IN OCCUPATIONAL DISEASE

A PRACTICAL GUIDE

MUNKSGAARD

Distributed in North, South and Central America by
Year Book Medical Publishers, Inc.

Symptoms and Signs in Occupational Disease
1st edition

Copyright © 1978 Munksgaard, Copenhagen
All rights reserved

Cover by Michael Clante

Composition: Grafisk Reklameproduktion

Printed in Denmark by Villadsen & Christensen, Hvidovre

ISBN 87-16-02668-3

Distributed in North, South and Central America,
Hawaii and Puerto Rico by
Year Book Medical Publishers, Inc.

ISBN 0-8151-2293-4

RECOMMENDED WARNING SIGNS CORRESPONDING TO THE LABELS ON THE COVER

WHO and EEC labelling (Recommendations by the WHO comittee on Transport
of Dangerous Goods). The numbers correspond to the labels on the cover.

Front Cover (WHO)

1   Explosives
2   Explosives of no significant hazard
3   Explosives. Very insensitive substances
4   Compressed non-inflammable gases
5   Inflammable liquids
6   Inflammable solids
7   Substances liable to spontaneous combustion
8   Substances which, in contact with water, emit inflammable gases
9   Oxidizing substances; Organic peroxides
10   Poisonous (toxic) substances; Danger groups I and II
11   Poisonous (toxic) substances; Danger group III
12   Danger infectious substances
13-15   Radioactive substances
15   Corrosives

Back Cover (EEC)

1 E   Explosive
2 O   Fire supporting (oxidizing)
3 F   Inflammable
4 T   Toxic
5 C   Corrosive
6 Xn   Unhealthy (lesser toxic)
7 Xi   Locally irritating without being corrosive

PREFACE

The present book is intended as a quick guide – an aide-mémoire – for physicians in cases where symptoms or symptom complexes do not conform with common clinical diseases or syndromes. The clinician handling a patient with inexplicable symptoms should remember Ramazzini's question: "What is your occupation?" Thus, the book should be regarded as a complement to the art of deducing a diagnosis from symptoms.

The author will welcome readers' criticisms and suggestions which may be og help if publishing a second edition. (see page 95).

Only the dose differentiate a poison from a remedy.

Paracelsus (1494-1541)

CONTENTS

SYMPTOMS AND SIGNS DUE TO CHEMICAL AND PHYSICAL INJURIES

Part I lists symptoms and signs which have been compiled from standard works on toxicology and occupational medicine. Due to authors' inconsistencies and vagueness it has been difficult and sometimes impossible to distinguish terms such as acute and chronic illness, or to differentiate between signs, e.g. sensor and motor polyneuropathia. Because of this we have sometimes been forced to put symptoms or signs under the same heading in an apparently illogical way, but the chief aim of the book is to raise a suspicion of occupational disease.

The listing has been done in alphabetical order without taking into account the shorter chemical prefixes namely: alpha-, beta-, bis-, ciphers, cis-, d-, gamma-, meta-, n-, nor-, N-, o-, orto-, para-, s-, sec- and ter-. Beta-naphthylamine is found under N, whereas trichloroethylene is listed under T.

The term chronic intoxication concerns symptoms which appear either as latent (i.e. a symptom-free interval after exposure to the agent) or as sequelae after an acute intoxication, or permanent, irreversible symptoms or reversible symptoms of long duration. To list the term "chronic" together with death may seem astonishing but means here delayed and/or inexplicable death. The exposure which caused death may otherwise have been forgotten.

Acute intoxication means initial and sometimes delayed symptoms (some hours after exposure).

As the aim of the book concerns occupational risks, acute oral poisoning has not been mentioned, as this – in industry – is nearly always either accidental or intentional (suicidal). In cases of poisoning by ingestion standard handbooks on acute, oral poisoning should be consulted.

Symptoms due to bacterial or viral infections and to psychological factors such as stress, etc. are not covered by this book; neither are the causes of allergic contact dermatitis, as highly specialized books dealing with this topic are already available.

An attempt to range symptoms according to importance or frequency has not been done, as this implies individual sensitivity and dose/time-response relationship.

When only the name of an element is mentioned, all its compounds should be considered as possible causes of the symptom.

Causes or active agents have been divided into three groups:
1. Agents with proven toxicity to man.
2. Agents with suspected, but not proven, toxicity to man; i.e. agents, whose toxicity is not generally accepted or subject to different opinions in literature.
3. The toxicity has only been proven in animal experiments.

Old-fashioned occupational stigmata such as "miners' knee" or "bakers' anaemia" have not been mentioned unless they are of particular interest.

Abdominal tenderness

Acute   *1* Carbon tetrachloride,

Abortion (abortus) see Embryonic development disorders

Accomodation disorders see Vision disorders

Achromatopsia see Vision disorders

Acidosis, metabolic

Acute   *1* Carbon monoxide,
Chronic *1* Acetone,
                 Dinitro-o-cresol, dinitrophenol, Methanol,

Acne see Skin dystrophia

Acoustic neuritis see Deafness and Vertigo

Acute yellow atrohpy see Liver disease

Adams-Stoke's attack see Arrythmia

Adiadochokinesis see Ataxia

Ageusia see Taste disorders

Agranulocytosis see Leucopenia

Air hunger see Dyspnoea

Albuminuria

Acute   *1* Dibutyl phtalate, Oxalic acid, Tellurium,
                 tetrachloroethane, thallium,
Chronic *1* Acetonitrile, arsine, Cadmium, carbon disulphide, carbon
                 tetrachloride, chlorotoluidine, Dioxane, Ethylene
                 chlorohydrin, Lead (inorganic), Mercaptans, Physical
                 effort (heavy), Vanadium,

Alcohol intolerance

Acute   *1* Butyraldoxim, Calciumcyanamide, Ethyleneglycol
                 dinitrate, Tetraethyl thiuram disulphide, TETD,
                 tetramethyl thiuram disulphide, tetramethyl thiuram
                 monosulphide, thiurams, TMTD, TMTM,
                 trichloroethylene,

Alopecia

Acute   *3* Trichlorobenzene,
Chronic *1* Arsenic, Chloroprene monomer, cyclophosphamide,
                 Hexamethyldisilane, Lead (inorganic), Mercury, Thallium
                 (after discolouration of hair),

Alveolitis see Lung fibrosis

Amaurosis see Blindness

Amblyopia see Blindness

Amenorrhoea

Chronic *1* Carbon disulphide, Lead,

Amnesia

Chronic *1* Mercury (inorganic), methyl chloride,

Anaemia including aplastic and haemolytic a.

Acute   *1* para-Aminosalicylic acid, 2-amino-5-sulfanilylthiazole,
                 Ethylene glycol, Methyl cellosolve (monomethyl ether),

1: Proven toxicity   2: Suspected toxicity

6

Paraquat (a herbicide), perchloryl fluoride, Stibine, Vanadium,

3 Ethyl silicate,

Chronic 1 Acrylonitrile, aminopterin, aniline, ankylostomiasis (mining), arsenic (organic), arsine, Benzene, Cadmium, carbon disulphide, carbon tetrachloride, cryolite, DDT, dinitrobenzenes, dinitrotoluene, dioxane, Ethyl acetate, Fluorides, Hexachlorocyclohexane (Lindane), Iodides, Klordane (organochlorine pesticide), Lead (inorganic), lindane (organochlorine pesticide), Manganese, methyl chloride, methyl glycol, Naphthalene, nitrobenzene, Phenyl hydrazine, potassium chlorate, pseudocumene, pyrocatechol, Tetrachloroethane, tetryl, thiocyanates, toluene, toluene diamines, Vinylchloride monomer, Xylenes,

2 Phosphine, Thiourea,

3 alpha-Aminoanthraquinone, Diacetone alcohol,

Analgesia

Acute 1 Dimethyl sulphate,

Angina pectoris see Chest pain

Angiospasm see Raynaud's phenomenon

Anhidrosis see Sweating, suppression of

Ankle drop see Polyneuropathia

Anorexia see also Weight loss

Acute 1 Benzanthrone, benzene, beryllium, Dinitrocresol, dinitrophenol, dioxane, Nitromethane, Organophosphate pesticides, Perchlorylfluoride, phosphine, polymethacrylate vapours, pyridine, Tetrachloroethane, tetraethyl lead, Vanadium,

Chronic 1 Aluminium, antimony, arsenic, Benzene, beryllium, Carbon disulphide, cresols, cyanides, Di-cyclo-heptadiene dibromide, dioxane, Ethylene dichloride, ethylene glycol, ethylene glycol dinitrate, ethyl ether, Fluorides, Guaiacol, Lead (inorganic), Manganese, mercury, methanol, methyl chloride, Nitrobenzene, Pentachlorophenol, phenol, phosphorous, Radiation (ionising), Tellurium, thallium, p-toluene sulfonyl chloride,

Anosmia including dys-, hyp- & parosmia

Acute 1. Formaldehyde, Hydrogen selenide, hydrogen sulphide, Phosgene, phosphorous oxychloride, Selenium, sulphuric acid,

Chronic 1. Benzene, benzine, butyl acetate, Cadmium, carbon disulphide, chalk dust, chromium, cyanides, Ethyl acetate, Hydrazine, Potash dust, Sulphur dioxide,

2. Cyclohexanone, Tetrahydrofurane,

Anoxaemia see Asphyxia

3: Toxicity only proven in animal experiments

Antabus effect

Acute   *1.*   n-Butyraldoxim, Calcium cyanamide, Tetramethyl thiuram disulphide, tetramethyl thiuram monosulphide, thiourams, trichloroethylene,

Anuria see Uraemia

Apathia see Psychiatric symptoms

Aphony see Laryngitis

Aplastic anaemia see Anaemia

Apnoea see Dyspnoea

Arrythmia of heart (including Bradycardia, ECG disorders, Palpitations, Tachycardia)

Acute   *1.*   Allyldibromide, arsine, Barium oxide, boranes, Carbon dioxide, carbon monoxide, chlorothene (1,1,1-trichloroethane), chlorotoluidine, cresols, N,N'-Di-sec-butyl-para-phenylenediamine, dimethyl sulphate, Electric shock, ethylene dichloride, Histamine, hydrazoic acid, Mercaptans, methanol, methyl acetate, Nitrous oxides, Parathion (organophosphate pesticide), Resorcinol, Tetraethyl and -methyl lead, trichloroethylene,

        2.   Fluoroacetic acid,
        3.   Fluorocarbones,

Chronic 2.   Dinitroglycol,

Ascites see Oedema, general

Asphyxia including Anoxaemia, Respiratory paralysis

Acute   *1.*   Aniline, Carbon dioxide, carbon monoxide, cotarnine chloride, cyclohexane, Diethyl aniline, dimethyl aniline, diphenylamine, Epichlorhydrin, ethylene, ethylene dichloride, ethyl ether, Gasoline, Heptachlor (organochlorine pesticide), hydrogen cyanide, hydrogen sulphide, Inert gases, Mercury, Noble gases, Organophosphate pesticides, Tetrachloroethane,

        3.   2,4-Dithiobiuret,

Asthenia see Tiredness

Asthma including Bronchospasm, Obstructive lung disease, Wheezing, see also Extrinsic allergic alveolitis

Acute   *1*   Acacia gum (printers' a.), acetic anhydride, allethrin, allyl isothiocyanate, aminoethylethanolamine, Chromium, cobalt (Hard Metal Disease), Dimethyl sulphate, Gum arabic (printers' a.), Piperazine, TDI (toluene diisocyanate), Vanadium pentoxide,

        2   Phtalic anhydride,

Chronic 1   Alfalfa meal, para-aminophenol, ammonium bichromate, Bicycloheptadiene dibromide, Chromates, Diazomethane, dichloroethyl ether, diethylenetriamine, Enzymes (proteolytic), ethylene oxide, extrinsic allergic alveolitis, Grain smuts, Hemp dust, MDI (diphenylmethane-4,4-di-isocyanate), Osmium, ozone, para-Phenylenediamine,

1: Proven toxicity   2: Suspected toxicity

phosgene, platinum (complex compounds), polyvinyl chloride (fumes, meat wrappers' a.), Saw dust, TDI (toluene diisocyanate), tetryl, trimethylbenzene, Vegetable dust, Wood dust,

    2 Acrolein, aluminium, Fluorides, Phosporous oxychloride,

Ataxia including Adia docho kinesis, Incoherent speech, Incoordination, Involuntary movements, Speech disorders, see also Staggering gait and Tremor

Acute   *1* Allyldibromide, Benzene, Carbon disulphide, cyclohexanol, Decompression sickness, Hydrogen cyanide, hydrogen sulphide, Methyl bromide, methyl chloride, Organic solvents, organophosphate pesticides, Pyrethrins, Toluene, trichloroethane,

Chronic 1 Acrylamide, anilines, Benzanthrone, Cyanides, Manganese, mercury (inorganic), Occupational cramps (e.g. writers' cramp), Thallium, TOCP (tri-orto-cresylphosphate),

    3 Ethylbenzene, Phosphine,

Bad taste see Taste disorders

Basophilia, basophilic granulation of leucocytes

Chronic 1 Aniline,

Basophilic punctuation of erythrocytes

Chronic 1 Lead (inorganic)
    2 Arsine,

Behavioural change see Psychiatric symptoms

Bilirubinaemia see Jaundice

Bitter taste see Taste disorders

Black urine see Urine discolouration

Bladder irritation see Miction disturbances

Blaesitas see Hoarseness

Blepharitis see Conjunctivitis

Blepharospasm see Myopathia

Blindness, amaurosis, amblyopia

Acute   *1* Cresol, Parathion, Vanadium,
Chronic 1 Coffee (coffee tasters), Methanol,
    2 Sodium aminophenol arsonate,

Blood coagulation defect see Thrombocytopenia

Blood disorders without specification

Acute   *1* Xylidine,
Chronic 1 Bicycloheptadiene dibromide,
    3 Diacetone alcohol, Germanium tetraphenyl,

Blue line of teeth

Chronic 1 Lead (inorganic), Mercury (inorganic),

Blurring of vision see Vision disorders

Bone marrow depression see Leucopenia

3: Toxicity only proven in animal experiments

Bone sclerosis see also Osteomalacia

Chronic 1 Cryolite, Fluorides,

Bradycardia see Arrythmia

Bronchitis

Acute 1 Acetaldehyde, acetic anhydride, acroleine, aldehydes, allyl alcohol, allyl chloride, allyl propyldisulphide, aluminium sulphate, aluminium carbide, ammonia, arsenic, Benzoyl chloride, benzoyl peroxide, bromide, butyl acetate, butyl glycol, n-butyl-isocyanate, butyl toluene, Cadmium, chlorine, chlordioxide, chloropicrine, cyanogen bromide, cyclohexanone, cyclotetramethylene oxide, Diazomethane, dibutylphtalate, dichloroethylene, dichloroethyl ether, dichlorohydrin, diethylene triamine, difluoromethane, dimethyl sulphate, dioxane, Ethyl acetate, ethyl alcohol, ethylamine ketone, ethyl bromide, ethylene bromide, ethylene oxide, ethyl-morpholine, ethyl silicate, Fluorine, fluoroform, fluorotrichloromethane, formaldehyde, furfural, Glycide aldehyde, 2-Heptadecyl-imidoazoline, heptane, cis-hexahydrophtalic anhydride, hexylene glycol, hydrazine, hydrazoic acid, hydrochloric acid, hydrofuramide, hydrogen azide, hydrogen chloride, hydrogen fluoride, hydrogen peroxide, Iodine, isoamyl acetate, isobornylthiocyanoacetate, isocyanates, isoprene, isopropyl ether, Methyl acetate, methyl bromide, 2-methyl-1-butanol, methyl ethyl ketone, methyl iso-butyl ketone, methyl propyl carbinol, methyl pyridine, monochlorbenzene, Nitric acid, nitrous oxides, n-nonane, Organophosphate pesticides, osmium tetroxide, oxalic acid, ozone, Pentanone-2, perchloroethylene, perfluoro-isobutylene, peroxides, phosphine, phosphorous oxychloride, phosphorous pentachloride, phosphorous pentoxide, phosphorous trichloride, phtalic anhydride, picoline, Selenium hydride, styrene (and fumes from polystyrene), sulphur chloride, sulphur dioxide, sulphuric acid, sulphur trioxide, TDI (toluene diisocyanate), tetrahydrofurane, tetranitromethane, Thomas' slag (basic slag) dust, trichloronitromethane, trifluorobromomethane, turpentine, tungsten, Vanadium, vinyl pyridine, Wolfram, Zinc chloride,

Chronic 1 Acetic acid, acroleine, Boranes, Cobalt, cyanides, Epichlorohydrin, Fluorides, formaldehyde, Guaiacol, gamma-Hexachlorocyclo-hexane, hydrogen sulphide, Inert dust, iron oxide, Lindane (organochlorine pesticide), Nitric acid, nitriles, Phenol, phtalic anhydride, platinum, pseudocumene, Sulphur, sulphur dioxide, sulphuric acid, Thomas' slag (basic slag) dust, Trimethylbenzenes,

    2 Phosphine,

Bronchospasm see Asthma

Cachexia see Anorexia and Weight loss

Cancer, urinary bladder,

Chronic 1 2-Acetylaminofluoride, 4-aminodiphenylmethane, aminotriphennylmethane, aniline, anthracene, Benzidine and salts, Coffee, aldol-alpha-Naphthylamine, beta-naphthylamine, Pentamethyl-para-fuchsin,

2 Polyoxyethylene stearate,

3 Diethylene glycol, 1-Naphthol-hydrochloride,

Cancer, bones

Chronic 1 Americium, Berkelium, Curium, Plutonium (Pu^{239}), Radium,

Cancer, ethmoidal sinuses

Chronic 1 Nickel carbonyl,

Cancer, liver (primary)

Chronic 1 Dimethylnitrosamine, Vinylchloride monomer,

2 Selenium, Thiourea,

3 Trichloroethylene,

Cancer, lungs

Chronic 1 Antimony, arsenic, asbestos, BCME (bis-chloromethyl ether), beryllium, Chromium (compounds OTHER THAN hydrogen-, sodium-, lithium-, ammonium-, cerium-, potassium- and rubidium mono- or dichromates and chromium anhydride), Dichloro-diethylsulphide, Iron ore, isopropyl oil, Lead, Methyl chloromethyl ether, mustard gas, Nickel, Oil (mineral), Plutonium (Pu^{238}), Radon (and radon daughters), Soot black, Uranium,

2 Carbamates, Formaldehyde, formalin, Glass fibers, Iron, Paraffin fumes,

3 Beryllium sulphate,

Cancer, nasopharyngeal (cavum nasi and paranasal sinuses)

Chronic 1 Isopropyl oil, Saw dust, soot black, Titanium, Wood dust, Zinc

Cancer, others (carcinogens and cocarcinogens)

Chronic 1 2-Acetamidofluorene, acetphenarsine, 2-acetylaminofluorene, acrylonitrile, 4-aminodiphenyl (p-xerylamine), antimony ore, arsenic, auramine, Benz-a-pyrine, benzidine and salts, buyo quid, Cacodyl oxide, cacodyl sulphide, calcium arsenide, calcium arsenite, calcium carbamate, carbon black, o-chlorine-p-nitroaniline, bis-chloromethyl ether, cutting oils, 2,4-Diamino-toluene, dibenzanthracene, dichloro-(2-chlorovinyl)arsine, dichloromethylarsine, diepoxides, dihydrogen potassium arsenate, dimetan (5,5-dimethyl-3-oxo-1-cyclohexen-1-yl-dimethyl-carbamate), dimethyl-amino-azo-benzene, N,N-dimethyl m-isopropylphenyl carbamate, dimethyl sulphate, dimetilane (2-dimethyl-carbamoyl-3-methyl-5-pyrazolyl dimethyl carbamate),

3: Toxicity only proven in animal experiments

11

dinitrosopiperazine, diphenylamine, disodium
acetoarsenate, disodium methane arsonate, DMBA (7,12-
dimethyl-benz-a-anthracene), dysprosium chromate,
Elocron (2-(1,3-dioxolan-2-yl)-phenyl-n-methyl carbamate,
equiline, ethyldichloro-arsine, Ferbam (ferric dimethyl
dithiocarbamate), ferric arsenate, ferric arsenide, ferric
dichromate, ferric ethylene-bis-dithiocarbamate, foot-soil,
Gallium arsenide, gasoline, gold ore, Hexamine-
chromium(III)-chloride, hexamine-nickel(II) nitrate,
hydrazine, hydrazine sulphate, hydrogen arsenide, Indium
arsenide, iron compounds, isolan (1-isopropyl-3-methyl-5-
pyrazolyl-dimethyl carbamate), isopropyl-N-(3-
chlorophenyl) carbamate, isopropyl oil, o-isopropyl-N-
phenyl carbamate, Kerosene, khaini, Lignite tar, lewisite,
Magnesium arsenate & arsenite, magnesium chromate,
maneb (manganeous ethylene-bis-dithio carbamate),
manganese cacodylate, mercuric chromate, mercuric
selenide, mercurous arsenide, mercurous chromate,
mercurous mono-hydrogen-o-arsenate, 4,4'-methylene-bis-
(2-chloroaniline), MOCA (3,3'-dichloro-4,4'-diamino-
diphenylmethane), Naphthol pitch, nickel compounds, o-
nitrobiphenyl, N-nitroso-dimethylamine, Paraffines,
phenetidines, phenylarsonic acid, phosphorous
pentaselenide, piperidinium, pentamethylene-dithio
carbamate, pyrolane, Rhizoctol (methyl arsenic sulphide),
Shale oil, Tin ore, tri-copper arsenide, trimethyl arsenic,
trinickel diphosphide, triphenyl arsenic, tryparsamide,
tsumacide, Urbacide,

2 Aldrine, 2,2-azonaphtalein, Bracken fern, butter yellow,
Cadmium, calcium cyclamate, calcium saccharin, calcium
selenide, calcium selenate, cedar wood oil, chlorinated
hydrocarbons, 1,2-Diethyl hydrazine, dimethyl-amino-azo-
benzene, Epichlorohydrin, Fish oils, Hydracrylic acid-
beta-lactone, Lard oil, lead (inorganic), Leather (chrome
tanned) Maleic hydrazide, manganese selenide, manganese
selenite, margarine emulsifiers, n-methyl-n-4-
dinitrosoaniline, 5-Nitro-2-n-propoxyaniline, 4-nitro-
quinoline-1-oxide, nitroso-benzyl, nitroso compounds, 2,2-
Oxydiethanol, 8-oxy-quinoline, Penicillium islandicum,
phenyl mercury-8-quinoline, polyamides, polyethylene,
polymethacrylates, polymethyl chlorosilicone, 8-Quinoline
(and compounds), Senecio alkaloids, sodium carboxy
methyl cellulose, sperm oil, Thioacetamide, tetraethyl lead,
trypan blue (esp. lymphoid tissue), tween 20-tris
(surfactans), Wool fat,

3. Acetic acid amine, acetylene urea, orto-amino-azotoluene,
CMME (chloromethyl-methyl ether), Diazomethane, 3,3'-
dichlorobenzidine, diethyl sulphate, dimethyl carbamide
chloride, dioxane, Ethionine (2-amino-4-(ethylthio)-butyric
acid), ethyl carbamate, ethylene oxide, ethylene imide,
Glycide aldehyde, Methyl chloromethyl ether, 1-Nitroso-2-

1: Proven toxicity   2: Suspected toxicity

naphthol, Propane sultone, beta-propriolactone, propylene-imine, propylene oxide, phenol, phenyl-mercury-8-quinolinol, SPAN, Trichloroethylene, Urethane, Vincyclohexene,

Cancer peritoneal

Chronic 1. Asbestos,
Cancer, prostatae

Chronic 1. Cadmium, cobalt,
Cancer, skin

Chronic 1. Amines, amino-diphenyls, 2-amino-1-naphthol, anthracene, arsenic, asphalt, Black wax, blast furnace tar, blue oil, bunker C fuel oil, BCME (bis-chloromethyl ether), Candle pitch, bis-chloromethyl ether, chloroprene monomer, coal tar, creosote, Mineral oil, 3-methylcholantrene, beta-Naphthylamine, Paraffin wax, PCBs (polychlorinated biphenyls and naphthalenes), petroleum waxes, pitch, phenantren, Ultraviolet light, Welding arcs,

2. Zinc chloride,

Cancer, thyroid

Chronic 1. Selenium, Thiourea,
Cardiac failure see Dyspnoea and Oedema, general

Caries see Dental erosions

Cartilage discolouration see Ochronosis

Cataract including Lens opacities

Acute 1. Electric shock, Infra-red light, IR-radiation, Lightning, Microwaves, Traumata (mechanical),

Chronic 1. Aromatic nitrocompounds, Cobalt, para-Dichlorobenzene, dinitro-o-cresol, dinitro phenol, Ionising radiation, Heat (= IR-light), Naphthalene, Selenium, Tellurium, Thallium, thorium,

3. Deka-hydronaphthalene, tetra-hydronaphthalene,

Catharsis see Diarrhoea

Cauliflower ear

Chronic 1. Professional boxing,
Central nervous system disorders without specification

Acute 1. Hydrogen sulphide,
Chronic 1. Methyl bromide, Thiocyanate,
Cephalalgia see Headache

Chalkosis see Vision disorders

Chest pain including Angina Pectoris, Chest Constriction, Chest discomfort, Chest tightness, Precordial pain, Retrosternal pain

Acute 1. Aniline, Beryllium, boranes, bromine, Cadmium, carbon disulphide, cobalt (Hard Metal Disease), Decompression sickness, diethyl aniline, dimethyl aniline, dimethyl sulphate, diphenyl amine, Ethyl benzene, Formaldehyde, Hydrogen cyanide, Iodine, iron pentacarbonyl,

3: Toxicity only proven in animal experiments

isocyanates, Mercury, metal fume fever, methyl cyanide, Nickel carbonyl, Organophosphate pesticides, ozone, Phosphine, polymer fume fever, Selenium,

Chronic 1. Acetonitrile, aluminium, Beryllium, Cotton dust (byssinosis), Dinitrophenol, Enzymes (proteolytic), ethylene chlorohydrin, Hydrogen sulphide, Osmium, Platinum (complex compounds), Sulphur dioxide, Vanadium,

Chills see Fever

Cholesterolaemia

Chronic 1. Carbon disulphide, Methylene chloride,

Cholinesterase low serum level

Chronic 1. Organophosphate pesticides,

Chorea see Ataxia

Choroiditis

Chronic 1. Iron dust,

Cirrhosis hepatis see Liver disease

Clubbing of fingers

Chronic 1. Asbestosis, Extrinsic Allergic Alveolitis,

CNS depression see Coma

Coagulation defect see Thrombocytopenia

Coeliac disease

Chronic 1. Accompanying Extrinsic Allergic Alveolitis (e.g. Farmers' lung),

Colics see Pains, abdominal

Collapse including Shock, Syncope, Fainting

Acute 1. Aniline, arsenic, arsine, Cadmium, cyanides, Decompression sickness, diethylaniline, dimethyl aniline, diphenyl amine, Histamine, hydrogen sulphide, Guaiacol, Histamine, hydrogen sulphide, Iron pentacarbonyl, Mercaptans, methyl dithiocarbamate (together with ethanol), Phenol, pyrethrins, Ricin,

Colour blindness see Vision disorders

Colour vision defect see Vision disorders

Coma including CNS-depression, Narcosis, Stupor, Unconsciousness

Acute 1. Acetaldehyde, acetone, acetylene, 2-amino-pyridine, anabasine (neonicotine), aniline, arnica (mountain tobacco), arsenic compounds, arsine, Benzene, boranes, Cadmium, carbon disulphide, carbon monoxide, carbon tetrachloride, chlorobenzenes, chloroform, chlorosulfonic acid, cresols, cyclohexane, cyclohexanol, cyclohexanone, cyclopentane, cyclopropane, Dichlorodifluoromethane, dieldrine, diethylaniline, 1,1-difluoroethane, dimethylaniline, dimethyl ether, dinitrobenzene, dioxane, diphenyl amine, Ethyl acetate, ethyl alcohol, ethyl

1: Proven toxicity   2: Suspected toxicity

bromide, ethyl chloride, ethylene dichloride, ethyl ether, ethyl fluoride, ethyl nitrite, Fluoroform, Guaiacol, Heptane, hydrogen cyanide, Inert gases, iron pentacarbonyl, iso-octane, isopropyl acetate, Kerosene, Mesityl oxide, methyl acetate, methyl bromide, methyl-isobutyl ketone, methyl chloride, methylene chloride, methyl iodide, methyl methacrylate, methyl nitrate, methyl nitrite, MIBK, Naphthalene, nickel carbonyl, nitroaniline, Octane, organic solvents, organochlorine pesticides, Pentanone-2, petroleum naphta, phenol, phosphine, pyridine, Ricinine, Styrene, sulphur dioxide, Tetraethyl lead, thallium, toluene, p-toluene-sulfonylchloride, trichloroethylene, trimethylene trinitramine, Vanadium, White spirit, Xylene,

2. Diphenyl ketene,

3. Alkyl amines, allyl glycidyl ether, Ethyl silicate, Monochloromonobromo methane, Nitrophenols,

Chronic 1. Acetonitrile, Ethylene, ethylene chlorhydrin, Glycol, Methanol, methyl bromide, methyl cyanide, monochlorobenzene.

3. Methylcyclopentadienylmanganese tricarbonyl,

Coma hepaticum see Liver disease

Confusion see Delirium

Conjunctivitis including Blepharitis, Corneal ulcer, Keratitis, Lachrymation, Photophobia, Pigmentation of Cornea, "Red eye", "Rose eye"

Acute 1. Acacia gum, acetaldehyde, acetic acid, acetic anhydride, acetone, acroleine, acrylamide, aldehydes, allyl alcohol, allyl chloride, allyl dibromide, allyl isothiocyanate, allylpropyldisulphide, ammonia, amyl acetate, amyl alcohol, apoatropine (atropamine), arc welding, arsenic, BAL (British Anti Lewisite), benzene sulphonyl chloride, benzine, benzoyl peroxide, benzyl alcohol, benzyl bromide, benzyl chloride, benzyl dichloride, beryllium, bis-1,4-bromacetoxy-2-butene, bromine, bromochloromethane, bromoform, butadienedioxide, butanol, butylacetate, butyl glycol, n-butyl isocyanate, Carbon (graphite and soot), carbon disulphide, cedar wood dust, chlorine, chloroacetophenone, chloroacetyl chloride, chloroform, chloroprene monomer, chlorosulfonic acid, chlorpicrine, coal tar, cobalt, colchicine, cresols, crotonaldehyde, cyanogen bromide, cyanogen chloride, cyclohexanone, cyclotetramethyleneoxide, Diacetone alcohol, dibromoethyl ether, dibutylphtalate, dichlorobenzene, dichloroethane, dichloroethylene, 2,2'-dichloroethyl ether, dichlorohydrin, dichloromethane, alpha-beta-dichloromethyl-ethyl ketone, 2,3-dichloro-1,4-naphtoquinone, dichloropropane, N,N-diethyl-m-toluamide, dimethyl-amino-ethyl methacrylate,

3: Toxicity only proven in animal experiments

dimethylcarbamide chloride, dimethyl formamide, dimethyl hydantoin formaldehyde resin, 2,3-dimethyl pentanol, dimethyl sulphate, dioxane, diphenylcyano-arsine, Epoxides, ethyl acetate, ethyl alcohol, ethyl amyl ketone, ethyl benzene, ethylenechlorohydrin, ethylene diamine, ethylene dibromide, ethylene dichloride, ethyl oxide, ethyl formate, ethylglycol acetate, ethyl-n-morpholine, ethyl silicate, Formaldehyde, formic acid, furfural, Gasoline, gum arabic, 2-Hepta-decyl-imido-azoline, hexafluoroacetone, hexylene glycol, hydrazine, hydrazoic acid, hydrofluoric acid, hydrogen azide, hydrogen cyanide, hydrogen fluoride, hydrogen peroxide, hydrogen selenide, hydrogen sulphide, N-hydroxy-ethyl-pyrrolidine, Iodine, iron dust, isobornyl-thiocyanate, isobutylenoxide, isophrone, isoprene, isopropanol, isopropylether, Ketene, Laser beam, lauroyl peroxide, MEK, metaldehyde, methanol mercury vapour lamps, MIBK, methyl acetate, methyl bromide, 2-methyl-1-butanol, methyl ethyl ketone, methyl ethyl ketone peroxide, methyl formate, methyl isobutyl ketone, methyl methacrylate, methyl propyl carbinol, methyl vinyl ketone, MIPA, monochlorbenzene, mono-isopropanol amine, morpholine, N-(alpha-(1-nitroethyl)-benzyl)-ethylene-diamine, Naphthalene, nitric acid, N-(alpha-(1-nitroethyl)-benzyl)-ethylene diamine, Organic solvents, osmium, oxalic acid, ozone, Pentamethyl-parafuchsin, pentanone-2, perchloroethylene, perfluoro-isobutylene, peroxides, N-(1-phenyl-2-nitropropyl)-piperazine, phosgene, phosphorous acid, phosporous oxychloride, phosphorous pentachloride, phosporous pentafluoride, phosphorous pentoxide, phosphorous trichloride, phtalic anhydride, pitch, potassium hydroxide, pyridine, Quinine, quinone, Resorcinol, ricin, ruthenium tetroxide, Selenium, selenium dioxide, sodium chloride, sodium hydroxide, sodium isopropylxanthate, solvents (organic), styrene (fumes from polystyrene), sulphur chloride, sulphur dioxide, sulphuric acid, sulphur monochloride, Tar dust, TDI, tetrachloroethane, tetrachloroquinone, tetrahydrofurane, tetranitromethane, thionyl chlorides, tin (organo-compounds), toluene diisocyanates, p-toluene-sulfonyl chloride, trichloroethane, trichloroethylene, trichloronitromethane, turpentine, Ultraviolet light, Vanadium, vinyl pyridine, vinyl toluene, Welding (arc), white spirit, Xylene, Zinc, zinc diethyl-dithio-carbamate, zinc dimethyl-dithio-carbamate,

Chronic 1. Acetic acid, acroleine, acrylamide, alfalfa meal, Butanol, Carbon tetrachloride, chloroprene monomer, coal tar, cresylic acid, cyanides, Enzymes (proteolytic), epichlorohydrin, epoxides, Gold, Hydrogen sulphide, hydroquinone, Iron ore, Lindane (gamma-hexachlorocyclohexane), Mining (Miners' nystagmus),

1: Proven toxicity   2: Suspected toxicity

Nitrogen mustard, Osmium, Phenol, pitch, Quinone, Saw dust, silver, sulphur dioxide, Tar, tetryl, Vanadium, Wood dust, Xylenes,

2. Lead, Tetramethyl silane,
3. Alkyl amines, Diphenyl-thio-carbazone, Ethylcyclohexanol,

Constipation

Chronic 1. Arsenic, Cadmium, Lead (inorganic), Mercury, Tellurium, thallium,

Convulsions including Cramps, Epileptic fits, Opistotonus, Terminal convulsions, Twitchings

Acute 1. Aconite, aldrine, 2-aminopyridine, anabasine (neonicotine), aniline, arsenic, Boranes, Carbon disulphide, chlordane, chlorobenzene, 2-chloro-4-dimethyl-amino-6-methyl-pyrimidine, cyclohexamine, Dichloroethylene, dieldrine, diethyl aniline, dimethyl aniline, dimethyl sulfoxide, diphenyl amine, Guaiacol, Heptachlor (organochlorine pesticide), hydrazine, hydrazoic acid, hydrofluoric acid, hydrogen azide, hyponatraemia (Stokers' cramp), Inert gases (symptoms of asphyxia), Lindane (gamma-hexa-chlorocyclohexane), Methyl bromide, methyl chloride, Naphthalene, nicotine, Organochlorine pesticides, organophosphate pesticides, Phenol, phosphine, pyrethrins, pyrocathecol, Resorcinol, ricinine, Styrene, Tetraethyl lead, thallium, p-toluene sulfonyl chloride, trimethylene-trinitramine, turpentine, Vanadium, White spirit,

2. Fluoroacetic acid,
3. Alkyl amines, Dichlorophene, diphenyl, Glycidyl aldehyde, Manganese tricarbonyl, methylcyclohexane, methylcyclopentadienyl, 2,2,4,4Tetramethyl-1,3-cyclobutanediol, tetramethylsuccinonitrile,

Chronic 1. Acetonitrile, arsenic, Mercury (inorganic), methanol, methyl cyanide, Tetrachloroethane, trimethylene-trinitramine,

3. Dieldrine,

Corneal oedema, haloes around light

Chronic 1. Dichloroethane, Maleic anhydride, morpholine, Osmium, Tetramethyl silane, Vanadium,

Corneal discolouration

Acute 1. Iodine (brown stain),

Corneal ulcers see Conjunctivitis and Keratitis

Coryza see Rhinitis

Cough severe, with or without expectoration, see also Bronchitis

Acute 1. Ammonia, amyl alcohol, Beryllium, boranes, butadienedioxide, Cadmium, chlorine, cobalt (Hard Metal Disease), cotton dust (mill fever), Diazomethane, dimethyl

3: Toxicity only proven in animal experiments

sulphate, dioxane, Ethylene oxide, Formaldehyde, Hydrazoic acid, hydrogen azide, hydrogen peroxide, Iodine, iron pentacarbonyl, isobutylene oxide, isocyanates, Mercury, metal fume fever, 2-methyl-1-butanol, methyl propyl carbinol, Nickel carbonyl, nitrous oxides, Phosgene, phosphine, phtalic anhydride, polymer fume fever, Selenium, sulphur dioxide, Tungsten, turpentine, Wolfram,

Chronic 1. Alfalfa meal, aluminium, Beryllium, Cadmium, cobalt, cotton dust (byssinosis), Diazomethan, Hydrogen sulphide, Iron Pentacarbonyl, Malt, Oxalic acid, Platinum (complex compounds),

Cramps: abdominal see Pains, abdominal

Cramps: muscular see Convulsions

Crepitations of lungs

Acute   1. Cobalt (Hard Metal Disease),

Cyanosis see also Methaemoglobinaemia

Acute   1. Ammonia, aniline, Barium oxide, beryllium, butyraldoxim (together with ethanol), Calcium cyanamide (together with ethanol), Decompression sickness, diethyl aniline, dimethyl aniline, dimethyl sulphate, dinitrobenzene, diphenyl aniline, Ethylene dichloride, Hydrogen selenide, Mercaptans, methyl bromide, monochlorobenzene, Nickel carbonyl, nitroaniline, nitrobenzene, Organophosphate pesticides, Perchlorylfluoride, Tetrachloroethane,

Chronic 1. Aniline, Chloronitrobenzene, chlorotoluidine, Diethyl aniline, dimethyl aniline, dinitrobenzene, dinitrocresol, dinitrophenol, diphenylamine, dinitrotoluene, Ethylenechlorohydrin, Extrinsic Allergic Alveolitis (e.g. Farmers' lung), Iron pentacarbonyl, Mannitol hexanitrate, nitroglycerin, Platinum (complex compounds), Resorcinol, TDI, TNT, toluenediisocyanate,

3. Alkyl amines,

Deafness, Hearing disorders, ototoxicity

Acute   1. Aconitine, anabasine (neonicotine), Methyl propyl carbinol, Noise,

Chronic 1. Carbon disulphide, Dinitrobenzene, Methanol, 2-methyl-1-butanol, methyl mercury, Noise,

2. Acetylene, aniline, Carbon monoxide, Hydrogen sulphide, Lead, Phosphorous, Silver,

Death

Acute   1. Acetonitrile, aconite, aconitine, aniline, arsenic, arsine, Benzene, berberine, beryllium, bromochloromethane, bromoform, Cadmium, carbon dioxide, carbon disulphide, carbon monoxide, carbon tetrachloride, chlordane, chlorine, cotarnine chloride, cyan, cyanogen bromide, cyanogen chloride, Decompression sickness, dichloro-(2-chlorovinyl)-arsine, dichloro-methyl-arsine, diethyl aniline, dimethyl aniline, dinitrobenzene, dinitrophenol, dioxane, diphenyl amine, Electric shock, epichlorohydrin, ethylene chlorohydrin, ethyl ether, Germanium hydride, guaiacol, Heptachlor (organochlorine pesticide), hydrazoic acid, hydrogen azide, hydrogen cyanide, hydrogen sulphide, Inert gases (asphyxia), Lewisite, Methanol, methyl bromide, methyl chloride, methyl mercury, Nickel carbonyl, nitrosyl chloride, Organophosphate pesticides, Paraquat, phenol, phosphine, Resorcinol, ricin, ricinine, Styrene, sulphur dioxide, Tetrachloroethane, tetraethyl lead, thallium,

3. Alkyl amines, Methyl cyclohexane,

Chronic 1. Antimony, Bicycloheptadiene dibromide, Dimethyl sulphate, Ethyleneglycol dinitrate, Ionising radiation, iron pentacarbonyl, Methyl chloride, Phenol,

Delirium including Confusion

Acute 1. Anabasine (neonicotine), Carbon disulphide, Dimethyl sulphate, Hydrogen sulphide, Methyl bromide, methyl chloride, methyl propyl carbinol, Tetraethyl lead, tetramethyl lead, thallium,

Chronic 1. Carbon disulphide, Ethylene dichloride, methyl bromide, 2-methyl-1-butanol, Sodium sulfocyanide, Tetrachloroethane,

Dementia see Psychiatric symptoms

Dental erosions including Caries, Discoloration, Necrosis

Chronic 1. Abrasive dust, acids and alkalies (fumes and aerosols), Bromides, Cadmium, cryolite, Flour dust, fluorides, Iodides, iron (e.g. nails held in mouth, carpenters), Manganese, mercury, Nickel, nitrocellulose, Strings (held in mouth), sugar dust, sulphur dioxide, Tartaric acid, Vanadium, X-rays,

2. Selenium,

Depilation see Alopecia

Depression, mental see Psychiatric symptoms

Dermatitis see Skin dystrophy

Dermatography

Acute   1. Vinyl chloride monomer,

Dermatosis see Skin dystrophy

Diaphoresis see Sweating

Diarrhoea including Purging

Acute   1. Aconite, para-aminosalicylic acid, arsenic, Benzyl alcohol, Cadmium, carbon tetrachloride, Dinitrophenol, Guanidine hydrochloride, Hydrocyanic acid, hydrogen sulphide, Lindane (gamma-hexa-chlorocyclohexane), Metal fume fever, methyl chloride, Nicotine, nitromethane, Organophosphate pesticides, Phosphine , polymer fume fever, pyrethrins, Ricin, Tellurium, thallium, TOCP, tri-orto-cresyl-phosphate, Vanadium,

3. Dichlorophene,

3: Toxicity only proven in animal experiments

Chronic 1. Acetonitrile, antimony, arsenic, Cadmium, chromium, cresols, Dinitrophenol, Guaiacol, Hydrogen sulphide, Ionising radiation, Lead (inorganic), Mercury, methyl cyanide, Phenol, Sodium sulfocyanide,

Diatesis haemorrhagica see Thrombocytopenia

Differential count, disorders or shift in, see Leucocytosis

Dimness of vision see Vision disorders

Diplopia

Acute 1. Methyl bromide,

Chronic 1. Methanol, methyl bromide, methyl chloride, Petrol fumes, pyridine,

Discolouration of nails see Nail dystrophy

Discolouration of teeth see Dental erosions

Dizziness see Vertigo

Drowsiness see Somnolence

Drunkenness see Psychiatric symptoms

Dry mouth see Pharyngitis

Dry throat see Pharyngitis

Dupuytren's contracture

Chronic 1. Pressure (local), Vibration,

Dysarthria see Ataxia

Dysbasia see Ataxia

Dysgeusia see Taste disorders

Dyspepsia see Gastro-intestinal disorders

Dyspnoea including Air hunger, Apnoea, Cardiac failure, Hyperpnoea, Jerky respiration, Laboured respiration, Respiratory depression, "Sighing respiration", Tachypnoea

Acute 1. Acrylonitrile, ammonia, aniline, Barium oxide, beryllium, boranes, bromine, butadiene dioxide, Cadmium, calcium cyanamide (together with ethanol), carbon dioxide, chlorobenzenes, cyanamide, Decompression sickness, N,N'-di-sec-butyl-paraphenylene-diamine, diethyl aniline, dimethyl aniline, dinitrobenzene, dinitrophenol, diphenylamine, Ethylene dichloride, ethylene oxide, Guaiacol, Hydrogen cyanide, hydrogen selenide, hydrogen sulphide, Inert gases (asphyxia), iron pentacarbonyl, isobutylenoxide, Mercury, methanol, methyl acetate, methyl chloride, methyl cyanide, Nickel carbonyl, nitrobenzene, nitrous oxides, Pentachlorophenol, phenol, phosphine, phosporous chlorides, pyrethrins, Ricinine, Sulphur dioxide, Thomas' slag (basic slag) dust, toluidines, tungsten, turpentine, Wolfram, Xylenes,

Chronic 1. Acetonitrile, aluminium, aniline, ankylostomiasis (mining), Beryllium, Cadmium, cobalt, cotton dust (byssinosis), Ethylene chlorohydrin, Iron pentacarbonyl, MDI (diphenyl-methane-4,4-diisocyanate), Resorcinol, Vanadium,

1: Proven toxicity   2: Suspected toxicity

      3. Alkyl amines, Methylcyclopentadienyl-manganese
           tricarbonyl,

Dysuria

Acute   *1.* Hydrogen sulphide,
Ebrietas see Psychiatric symptoms

ECG-disorders see Arrythmias

Edema see Oedema

Emaciation see Anorexia and Weight loss

Embryonic development disorders fetal defects, Stillbirths

Chronic 1. Aminopterin (4-aminopteroyl-glutamic acid), Carbon
           monoxide, chloroquine, Dimethyl formamide,
           dimethylnitrosamine, Halothane, hypoxia (high altitudes),
           Iodides, ionising radiation, Lead, Mercury (organic),
           Tetramethyl thiuram disulphide, tetramethyl thiuram
           monosulphide, thiouracil derivatives, TMTD, TMTM,

      2. Epichlorohydrin, Hexachlorophene, Methylene chloride,
          methyl-ethyl-ketone-peroxide,

      3. Diethylstilbestrol, Epichlorohydrin, ethyleneglycol-
          monomethyl ether,

Emphysema, pulmonary

Chronic 1. Aluminium oxide, Bauxite, beryllium, Cadmium,
           Dichlorethyl ether, Fluorides, Phosgene, Quartz
           (crystalline), Thomas' slag (basic slag)
      2. Manganese, Nitrous oxides, TDI, toluene diisocyanate,

Emphysema, subcutaneous

Acute   *1.* Caisson disease, Decompression sickness, dimethyl
           sulphate, Grease gun injury,

Chronic 1. Phosgene,
Encephalopathia organic cerebral lesion

Chronic 1. Boxing (professional), Lead (inorganic), Styrene monomer,
           Trimethyl-bismuthine,
Encephalosis see Psychiatric symptoms

Eosinophilia

Acute   *1.* Tellurium, thallium,
Chronic 1. Aluminium,
Ephidrosis see Sweating

Epilepsia, epileptic fits see Convulsions

Epiphora see Conjunctivitis

Epistaxis

Acute   *1.* Beryllium, Oxalic acid, Selenium, Vanadium,

Chronic 1. Benzene, Carbon tetrachloride, Enzymes (proteolytic),
           Hexamethyl-para-rosaniline. Phosphine, phtalic anhydride,
           Tetranitromethyl aniline, tetryl, trimethyl benzenes,
           Xylenes,

Erethismus see Psychiatric disorders

Erythema see Flush and Skin dystrophy

3: Toxicity only proven in animal experiments

Erythrocytosis see Polycythaemia

ESR, raised, Erythrocyte Sedimentation Rate

Chronic 1. Cadmium, Extrinsic Allergic Alveolitis (e.g. Farmers' lung),

Euphoria including Excitement, Exhilaration

Acute 1. Benzene, boranes, Hydrogen sulphide, Organic solvents, oxygen (divers, hyperbaric chambers), Methyl bromide, methyl chloride, Toluene,
 3. Alkyl amines,

Chronic 1. Carbon disulphide, Hydrogen sulphide,

Excitement see Euphoria

Exhilaration see Euphoria

Expectoration see Bronchitis

Extrapyramidal symptoms

Acute 1. Hydrogen sulphide, Tetraethyl lead,
 2. Boranes,

Chronic 1. Acrylamide, Carbon disulphide, carbon monoxide, Lithium, Manganese, mercury (inorganic), methanol, methyl mercury, Tellurium, thorium,

 2. Sulphur dioxide,

Fainting see Collapse

Fatigue see Tiredness

Fatty degeneration of liver see Liver disease

Fetal defects see Embryonic development disorders

Fever including Chills, Hyperthermia, see also Shivering

Acute 1. Boranes, Cadmium, cotton dust (mill fever), Dimethyl sulfoxide, dinitrocresol, dinitrophenol, Extrinsic Allergic Alveolitis (e.g. Farmers' lung), Hydrazoic acid, hydrogen azide, Ionising radiation, Manganese, mercury, metal fume fever, methyl bromide, methyl chloride, Naphtalene, nickel carbonyl, Polymer fume fever, Tetrachloroethane, Zinc oxide,
 2. alpha-Naphthyl-isothiocyanate, Zinc stearate,
 3. Nitrophenols,

Chronic 1. Dinitrobenzene, dinitro-o-cresol, dinitrophenol, Ionising radiation, iron pentacarbonyl, Lanthanons ("Rare Earths"), Malt,

Fibrosis pulmonum see Lung fibrosis

Flush of skin including Vasodilatation

Acute 1. Acrylonitrile (esp. face), aniline, arsenic, Benzene, Calcium cyanamide (together with ethanol), carbon disulphide, carbon monoxide, cyanamide, Decompression sickness, N,N'-di-sec-butyl-para-phenylene-diamine, diethyl aniline, dimethyl aniline, diphenyl amine, Histamine, hydrazoic acid, IR-light, Trichloroethylene,

1: Proven toxicity   2: Suspected toxicity

Foetor ex ore including Garlic odour of breath

Acute 1. Acetone, Hydrogen cyanide, hydrogen selenide, Isopropanol, Methanol, Phosporous, Selenium, Tellurium,

Chronic 1. Arsine, Cacodylic acid, Hydrogen sulphide, Selenium, Tellurium,

Fractures, spontaneous see Osteomalacia

Fractures vertebral

Acute 1. Electric shock,
Funnel chest pectus excavatus

Chronic 1. Shoemakers,

Garlic odour of breath see Foetor ex ore

Gastritis see Gastro-intestinal disturbances and Nausea

Gastro-intestinal disturbances, non-defined.

Acute 1. Acetylene, adiponitrile, armica (mountain tobacco), arsenic, arsine, Benzanthrone, berberine, Calcium iodobehenate, carbon disulphide, Dichlorohydrin, dimethylformamide (esp. gastritis), dioxane, Fluorine, Hydrochloric acid, Lindane (gamma-hexachloro-cyclohexane), Methanol, Naphthalene, nitrobenzene, 2-nitropropane, Organic solvents, organophosphate pesticides, Parathion, PCBs (polychlorinated biphenyls and naphthalenes), pyridine, pyridine methanol, Selenium, Tetraethyl and -methyl lead, tetramethylene cyanide,

Chronic 1. Ankylostomiasis (mining), antimony compounds, Carbon disulphide, chromium, cryolite, Ethylene dichloride, Guaiacol, Hydrogen sulphide, Mercury, Organic solvents, PCBs, phenol, phenylhydrazine, phosporous, polychlorinated biphenyls and naphthalenes, Selenium, Tellurium, tetryl, TNT, TOCP, trinitrotoluene, tri-orto-cresyl-phosphate,

2. Phosphine, Triethylene melamine,

Glucosuria

Acute 2. Methyl propyl carbinol,
Chronic 2. Carbon monoxide,
3. Diphenylthiocarbazone, 2-methyl-1-butanol,
Goiter see Thyroid enlargement

Giddiness see Vertigo

Gingivitis see also Blue line, Yellow line of teeth

Chronic 1. Antimony, arsenic, Bismuth, Cadmium, Lead (inorganic), Mercury,

Glossitis, glossalgia

Chronic 1. Arsenic, Enzymes (proteolytic), Selenium,
Granulopenia see Leucopenia

Green tongue

Chronic 1. Vanadium,

3: Toxicity only proven in animal experiments

Haematemesis

Acute 1. Arsenic, Cadmium, Methyl cyanide, Selenium,
Chronic 1. Acetonitrile, Benzene, Carbon tetrachloride,
Haematuria see Haemoglobinuria

Haemoglobinaemia see Haemolysis

Haemoglobinuria including Haematuria

Acute 1. 2-Amino-5-sulfanilylthiazole, arsine, Chlorobenzene,
Dioxane, Naphthalene, Stibine,

Chronic 1. Aniline, Carbon tetrachloride, chlorotoluidine, Diethyl
aniline, dimethyl aniline, diphenyl amine, Methyl chloride,
Phenylhydrazine, Toluidines,
Haemolysis including Haemoglobinaemia

Acute 1. 2-Amino-5-sulfanilylthiazole, aniline, arsine, Benzidine,
Copper compounds, Diethyl aniline, dimethyl aniline,
diphenyl amine, Germanium hydride, Helvellic acid,
hydrazin, Nitrobenzene, Ricin, Tellurium tetrahydrogen,

Chronic 1. Acetylhydrazine, aniline, Lanthanons ("Rare Earths"),
lead, Manganese, Phenothiazine, Tetrachloroethane, TNT,
toluenediamines, trinitrotoluene,

Haemolytic anaemia see Anaemia

Haemopoietic disturbances see Blood disorders and
Thrombocytopenia

Haemoptysis

Acute 1. Beryllium, Nickel carbonyl, Phosporous chlorides,
Thomas' slag (basic slag) dust, Vanadium,

Chronic 1. Extrinsic Allergic Alveolitis (e.g. Farmers' lung),
Haemorrhagia

Acute 1. Nitrous oxides (cerebral h.), Petroleum naphta (in "vital
organs"),

Chronic 1. Methyl chloride (in intestinal tracts, lungs, meninges),
Hair discolouration see Skin pigmentation

Hair disorders see Alopecia

Hallucinations see Psychiatric symptoms

Haloes round lights see Corneal Oedema

Headache

Acute 1. Acetaldehyde, acetic acid, acetone, acetylene,
acrylonitrile, 2-aminopyridine, amyl acetate, amyl alcohol,
amyl nitrite, aniline, arsenic, arsine, Benzene, benzine,
benzyl alcohol, butadiene dioxide, butylnitrite, Cadmium,
calcium cyanamide (together with ethanol), carbon
disulphide (esp. frontal headache), carbon monoxide,
carbon tetrachloride, cotton dust (mill fever), cresols,
cyclohexanol, Dibutylphtalate, dichloromethane,
dieldrine, diethyl aniline, dimethyl aniline, dinitrobenzene,
dioxane, diphenyl amine, diphenylchloroarsine, dynamite,
Ethylamine ketone, ethylene chlorohydrin, ethylene glycol
dinitrate, ethylene oxide, Guaiacol, Histamine, hydrazoic

acid, hydrocyanic acid, hydrogen cyanide, hydrogen
sulphide, Isoamyl acetate, isobutyl amine, isometheptene,
isobutyleneoxide, Kerosene, Lindane (gamma-
hexachlorocyclohexane), Mannitol hexanitrate,
mercaptans, metal fume fever, methyl acetate, methyl
bromide, 2-methyl-1-butanol, methyl chloride, methyl
nitrate, methyl propyl carbinol, Naphthalene, nickel
carbonyl, nitroaniline, nitroglycerin, Organic solvents,
organochlorine pesticides, oxalic acid, ozone,
Pentaerythritol tetranitrate, PETN, petroleum naphta,
phenol, phosphine, phtalic anhydride, polymer fume fever,
polymethyl methacrylate vapours, propylene oxide,
pyrethrins, pyridine, Stibine, styrene, Toluene, p-toluene
sulfonyl chloride, toluidines, trichloroethane,
trichloroethylene, trinitromethane, Vinyl chloride
monomer, White spirit,

Chronic 1. Acroleine, amyl alcohol, antimony, arsine, Boranes, boron
hydrides, Carbon disulphide, chloroform, cresols,
cyanides, Dinitrobenzenes, dinitrophenol, Enzymes
(proteolytic), ethylene chlorohydrin, extrinsic allergic
alveolitis, Guaiacol, Hydrogen cyanide, hydrogen sulphide,
Lanthanons ("Rare Earths"), Malt, manganese, mercury,
methanol, methyl chloride, microwaves, mining (miners'
nystagmus - occipital h.), monochlorobenzene,
Nitrobenzene, Osmium, Phenol, Selenium, Tellurium,
trimethyl-benzene,

  2. 2-Amino-thiazole, Carbon monoxide, Germanium, Phenyl-
mercaptan,

Hearing disorders see Deafness

Heart disease see also Arrythmias

Acute   1. Boranes,
Chronic 1. Antimony, Carbon disulphide, Methylene chloride,
Tetrachloroethane, Xylenes,

Hem- see Haem-

Hepatitis see Liver disease

Hepatomegalia see Liver disease

Hepatorenal syndrome see Liver disease and Kidney disease

Hiccup

Acute   1. Boranes, boron hydrides, butadiene dioxide, isobutylene
oxide,

Hoarseness see Laryngitis

Hyperaesthesia see Paraesthesia

Hyperazotaemia see Uraemia

Hypercalcuria

Chronic 1. Beryllium,
Hypercholesterolaemia see Cholesterolaemia

3: Toxicity only proven in animal experiments

Hyperglucaemia

Acute *1.* Pentachlorophenol,
Hyperhidrosis see Sweating

Hyperkeratosis see Skin dystrophia

Hyperpnoea see Dyspnoea

Hypersalivation see Salivation

Hypertension

Acute *1.* Carbon monoxide, Vanadium,
Chronic 1. Cadmium, carbon disulphide, coffee (coffee tasters),
        Dimethylformamide, Lead (inorganic), Mercury,

      2. Heavy metals, heat, Microwaves, Noise,

Hyperthermia see Fever

Hypoaesthesia see Paraesthesia

Hypoglucaemia

Chronic 3. Ethylene dichloride,
Hypoprothrombinaemia see Thrombocytopenia

Hyposmia see Anosmia

Hypotension

Acute *1.* Amyl nitrite, Butyl nitrite, Calcium cyanamide (together
        with ethanol ingestion), cyanamide, Dinitroglycol,
        Ethylene glycol dinitrate, ethyl nitrite, Histamine,
        Mannitol hexanitrate, Ozone, Pentaerythritol tetranitrate,
        PETN, polymethyl methacrylate vapours, propyl-nitrate,
        propyl nitrite, Sodium nitroprusside, Tetra ethyl and
        methyl lead,
Chronic 1. Ammonium nitrate, Benzanthrone, Dinitro-o-cresol,
        dynamite, Nitrites, nitroglycerin, Resorcinol,

Hypothermia

Acute *1.* Berberine, Guaiacol, Phenol, Tetra ethyl and methyl lead,
Chronic 1. Resorcinol,
Icterus see Jaundice

Impotence

Acute *1.* Carbon monoxide,
Chronic 1. Benzanthrone, benzine, Carbon disulphide, carbon
        monoxide, Hydrocarbons, Mercury, microwaves,

Incoherent speech see Ataxia

Incontinentia urinae see Miction disturbances

Incoordination see Ataxia

Influenza simulating

Acute *1.* Farmers' lung, Metal fume fever, Polymer fume fever,
Insomnia see also Psychiatric symptoms

Acute *1.* Tetraethyl lead, trimethylenetrinitramine,
Chronic 1. Antimony, Cadmium, carbon monoxide, Lead (inorganic),
        Mining (miners' nystagmus), Nitrous oxides,

Involuntary movements see Ataxia

Iridocyclitis

Chronic 2. Cedar wood dust,

Irritability see Psychiatric symptoms

Irritation of nose see Rhinitis

Ischidrosis see Sweating

Itching of skin

Acute 1. Acridine, Cyanides, Decompression sickness, dimethyl sulfoxide, Sulfuryl chloride,

Chronic 1. Acrylonitrile, ankylostomiasis (mining), arsenic, Cobalt ("carboloy itch"), Dogger Bank Itch (sea-chervil),

Jaundice, bilirubinaemia

Acute 1. Acrylonitrile, para-amino-salicylic acid, aniline, arsine, Boranes, boron hydrides, Diethyl aniline, diisocyanates, dimethyl aniline, dinitrophenol, diphenylamine, Paraquat, Stibine,

Chronic 1. Aniline, antimony, arsenic, arsine, Carbon tetrachloride, Dinitrobenzenes, Ethylene dichloride, Methylene dianiline, PCBs, phosporous, polychlorinated biphenyls and naphthalenes, Tetrachloroethane, TNT, toluenediamines, p-toluene sulfonyl chloride, trinitrotoluene,

3. cis-Dichloroethylene, Ethylenechlorobromide,

Jerky respiration see Dyspnoea

Kakogeusis see Bad taste

Keratitis including Corneal ulcers, Keratoconus

Acute 1. Acids, alkalies, ammonia, Butanol, Dimethyl-phosphoro-chloride-thionate (DMPCT), Ethylene dibromide, ethylene imine, ethylene oxide, Glyodine, Helvellic acid, cis-hexa-hydrophtalic anhydride, hydroquinone, Isopropanol, Maleic anhydride, mesityl oxide, alpha-Naphtol (even injury to lens), Potassium permanganate, Quinone, Sodium hydroxide, Soman (a nerve gas), styrene monomer, Tabun (a nerve gas), tetryl, thionyl chloride, tin (organocompounds), toluene,

2. Ethylene dichloride, Methylene chloride,

Chronic 1. Cedar wood dust, chromates, copper (metallic), Dichloroethane, Hydrogen sulphide, orto-Methyl silicate, Osmium, Quinone, Strontium hydroxide,

3. Ethylene imine, Germanium tetrachloride, Isophorone,

Keratoconus see Keratitis

Kidney disease, parenchymatous see also Albuminuria

Acute 1. Boranes, boron hydrides, Carbon tetrachloride, Dimethyl sulphate, dinitro phenol, dioxane, Heptachlor, Mercury, methyl bromide, methyl chloride, methyl iodide, alpha-Naphtol, 2-nitropropane, Organochlorine pesticides, Ricinine, Thallium, turpentine,

3: Toxicity only proven in animal experiments

2. Hydrofuramide, Metaldehyde,

Chronic 1. Allethrin, Beryllium, boranes, boron hydrides, butyltoluene, Cadmium, chloroform, cresol, cresylic acid, 2,4-Dichlorophenoxi acetic acid, dimethyl sulphate, dinitrobenzene, dinitrocresol, dioxane, DMDT (v.i.), Electric shock (myoglobinaemia), epichlorohydrin, ethyl bromide, ethylene dibromide, ethylene dichloride (hepatorenal syndrome), Guaiacol, Hydrazoic acid, hydrogen azide, Iron pentacarbonyl, Lead (inorganic), Methoxychlor (DMDT), methyl chloride, Pentachlorophenol, phenol, phenylhydrazine, pyridine, Tetrachloroethane, trifluoro-chloroethylene, turpentine, Uranium, Vinyl toluene,

2. Chlorobenzenes, Dichloropropane, Ethylene chlorohydrin, Hydrazine, Metaldehyde, methylcyclohexanone, Phenylhydrazine, Tetramethyl silane, turpentine,

3. Allyl chloride, amides (unsaturated & N-subtituted), alpha-amino-anthraquinone, Butyl glycol, Cyclotetramethylene oxide, Diacetone alcohol, dichlorobenzene, 2,2'-dichloroethyl ether, 1,2-dichloropropane, 1,3-dichloropropene, Ethyl chloride, Hexafluoro-dichlorocyclopentene, Isophrone, Lead stearate, Manganese cyclopenta-dienyl-tricarbonyl, mesityl oxide, methyl acrylate, methylal (methylene dimethyl ether), Nitroethane, nitrophenols, ter-Phenyls, TCPPA,. tetrahydrofurane, tetrahydronaphthalene, 2-(2,4,5-trichlorophenoxi)-propionic acid & compounds, triethanolamine,

Kidney stones see Stones, renal

Laboured breathing see Dyspnea

Labyrinthitis see Vertigo

Lachrymation see Conjunctivitis

Langour see Tiredness

Laryngitis including Aphony, Hoarseness

Acute 1. Arsenic, Dimethyl sulphate, Phtalic anhydride, Thomas' slag (basic slag) dust,

Chronic 1. Cyanides, Occupational disease (as in actors, clergymen), Phtalic anhydride,

Laryngospasm, laryngo-oedema

Acute 1. Hydrochloric acid,

Lassitude see Tiredness

Laughter, uncontrollable

Chronic 1. Manganese,

Lens opacity see Cataract and Keratitis

Lethargy see Somnolence

Leucocytosis including Lymphocytosis "shift in differential count"

Chronic 1. Hydroquinone monomethyl ether,

1: Proven toxicity   2: Suspected toxicity

Leucoderma see also Skin pigmentation

Acute *1.* Acrylonitrile, Dimethyl sulphate, dioxane, Electric shock, ethylene dichloride, ethylene glycol monomethyl ether, Metal fume fever, Polymer fume fever, Tellurium,

        3. Ethyl silicate,

Chronic 1. Antimony, Benzene, boranes, boron hydrides, Dimethyl formamide, Ethyl acetate, ethylene dichloride, Methyl chloride, Phtalic anhydride, Thallium,

        2. Organic solvents,

Leucopenia including Agranulocytosis, Bone marrow depression

Acute *1.* Benzidine, Dichloro-diethyl sulphide, Ionising radiation, Mustard gas,

Chronic 1. 4-Amino-folic acid, aminopterin, aminopyrine, Benzene, Carbon tetrachloride, cyclophosphamide, Dibenzyl-chloro-ethyl amine, dicycloheptadiene bromide, dinitrobenzene, dinitrophenol, Ethyl carbamate, Lindane (gamma-hexachloro-cyclohexane), Manganese, Toluene, Urethane, Xylenes,

        2. Dinitrophenol, alpha-Naphthyl-thiourea, Thiourea, triethylene melanine,

        3. Glycidyl aldehyde, Mesitylene (1,3,5-trimethyl benzene),

Leukaemia

Chronic 1. Benzene, para-Dichlorobenzene, Ionising radiation, Plutonium,

        2. Carbamates, Toluene,

Listlessness see Psychiatric symptoms

Liver disease including Acute yellow atrophia, "Chemical hepatitis", Enlarged liver, Fatty degeneration, Hepatomegalia, Hepatorenal syndrome, Parenchymatous liver damage, Cirrhosis hepatis, see also Jaundice

Acute *1.* Boranes, boron hydrides, bromochloromethane, Chlordane (organochlorine pesticide), 4,4-Diaminophenylmethane, dimethyl sulphate, diphenyl, Ethylene dibromide, Heptachlor (organochlorine pesticide), hexachloronaphthalene hydrazine, Methylene dianiline, Nickel carbonyl, 2-nitropropane, PCBs, polychlorinated naphthalenes and biphenyls, Ricinine, Tetranitromethane,

        2. Diisocyanates, Hydrofuramide, Metaldehyde,

Chronic 1. Allethrin, d-amyl bromide, antimony, Benzanthrone, benzene-sulphonyl-chloride, beryllium, boranes, Bordeaux mixture (vineyard sprayers), boron hydrides, bromofor, butyl toluene, Carbon tetrachloride, chloroform, cresols, Dimethyl formamide, dimethyl nitrosamine, dimethyl sulphate, dinitrobenzenes, dinitrocresol, dinitrophenol, dinitrotoluene, dioxane, diphenyls, Ethanol (e.g. wine tasters), ethyl bromide, ethylene dichloride (hepato-renal

3: Toxicity only proven in animal experiments

symdrome), Guaiacol, Hydrazoic acid, hydrogen azide, Iron pentacarbonyl, isopropanol (synergistic with other solvents), isopropylacetate, Methyl chloride, Naphthalene, nitroaniline, nitrobenzene, Paraquat, pentachlorophenol, phenol, phenothiazine, paraphenylenediamine, phenylhydrazine, pyridine, Styrene monomer, Tetrachloroethane, tetranitromethane, TNT, toluene diamines, trifluorochloroethylene, Uranium, Vinyl chloride monomer, vinyl ether, vinyl toluene,

2. Chlordane (organochlorine pesticide), chlorobenzenes, cresol, Dichloropropane, Guaiacol, Hydrazine, Methyl cyclohexanone, Phenol, Selenium, Toluene, 2,4-toluene-diisocyanate (TDI), Xylidine,

3. Acetylhydrazine, allyl chloride, amides (unsaturated and N-substituted), alpha-aminoanthraquinone, Butyl glycol, Cyclotetramethylene oxide, Diacetone alcohol, dichlorobenzene, cis-dichloroethylene, 2,2-dichloroethylene ether, 2,4-dichloro-phenoxyacetic acid, 1,2-dichloropropane, 1,3-dichloropropene, Ethyl chloride, ethylene chlorobromide, ethylidene chloride, Furfural, Heptachlor (organochlorine pesticide), hexachlorodiphenyl oxide, hexachloroethane, hydrogen selenide, Maleic hydrazide, mesityl oxide, methylal (methylenedimethyl ether), nitrodimethyl amine, nitroethane, nitrophenols, Phenothioxin, ter-phenyls, Tetrahydrofurane, thioacetamide, 2-(2,4,5-trichlorophenoxy)-propionic acid and compounds, triethanolamine,

Locked jaw see Trismus

Lung abscess

Chronic 1. Phosgene,

Lung disease without specifications

Acute 1. Telluriumhexafluoride,
Chronic 3. Hexafluoro-dichloro-cyclopentene, Methyl acrylate, methylal (methylenedimethyl ether), Silica (amorphous),

Lung fibrosis including Fibrosing alveolitis, Pneumoconiosis

Acute 1. Paraquat (a herbicide),
Chronic 1. Aluminium, asbestos, Barium, beryllium, Coal, cobalt (Hard Metal Disease), cryolite, Extrinsic Allergic Alveolitis (sequelae), Fluorides, Graphite, Iron, Lanthanons ("Rare Earths"), Mica, Quartz (crystalline), Thorium, tin, Vanadium, Zirconium,

2. Enzymes (proteolytic), Ozone, TDI (toluene diissocyanate), tungsten, Wolfram,

Lymphadenitis, enlarged lymphnodes

Acute 1. Dichloro-diethyl-sulphide, Mustard gas,
Chronic 1. Resorcinol,

Lymphocytosis see Leucocytosis

Lymphopenia

Chronic 1. Ionising radiation,

Mania see Psychiatric symptoms

Marasmus see Anorexia and Weight loss

Melaena

Acute 1. Arsenic,

Melancholia see Psychiatric symptoms

Menstruation disorders

Chronic 1. Xylenes,

Metallic taste see Taste disorders

Metastases of cancer simulating skeletal m.

Chronic 1. Cryolite, Fluorides,

Methaemoglobinaemia

Acute 1. Dinitrobenzene, Ethyl nitrite, Hydroxyl amine, Nitroaniline, nitrobenzene, 2-nitropropane, Perchlorylfluoride, potassium perchlorate,

Chronic 1. para-Aminophenol, aniline, Bromates, Chlorates, chloro-nitrobenzenes, Diethyl aniline, dimethyl aniline, dinitrobenzene, dinitrotoluene, dynamite, diphenyl amine, Glycerol trinitrate, Mannitol hexanitrate, 2-methyl-1-butanol, methyl propyl carbinol, metol, Nitrites, nitroglycerin, Propyl nitrate, Resorcinol, Tetranitromethane, TNT, trinitrotoluene,

3. Nitrophenols,

Micrographia see Extrapyramidal symptoms

Miction disturbances including Bladder irritation, Incontinence, Retention

Acute 1. Ammonia (retention), aniline (incontinence), Carbon tetrachloride, Diethyl aniline, dimethyl aniline, diphenyl amine, Methyl bromide, Toluidines,

Chronic 1. Acrylamide, Mercury, Trichloroethylene,

Milkman syndrome see Osteomalacia

Miosis

Acute 1. Glycidaldehyde, Nitrobenzene, Organophosphate pesticides,

Muscular disorders see Myopathia

Mydriasis

Acute 1. Aconite, atropine, Diethylamino-ethylchloride, dimethyl-aminoethylchloride, dinitrophenol, Methyl bromide, Tetra ethyl and methyl lead,

Myopathia including Blepharospasm, Fasciculations, Pains, Tenderness, Twisting, Weakness, Convulsions, Cramps, Myocarditis

Acute 1. Ethylene chlorohydrin, Guaiacol, Metal fume fever, Organophosphate pesticides, Phenol, polymer fume fever, Sulphuryl fluorides, Tetraethyl lead, trichloroethylene,

3: Toxicity only proven in animal experiments

Chronic 1. Aniline, antimony, Boranes, boron hydrides, Ethylene chlorohydrin, Lead (inorganic), Mining (Miners' nystagmus – blepharospasm), Thallium (heart muscle and calves of legs),

2. Carbon disulphide, carbon monoxide (primary myonecrosis),

3. Cesium,

Myoglobinaemia

Acute 1. Physical effort (heavy),
Chronic 1. Electric shock,

Nail dystrophia including Loss of nails, Discolouration

Acute 1. Hydrofluoric acid, Selenium dioxide (red discolouration, tenderness of nail beds),

Chronic 1. Amethocane, aminoethylethanol amine (aluminium soldering flux), arsenic, bromine, butanol, para-tert-butyl phenol, Chloroprene monomer, cosmetics, Epoxides, Formalin, Onions and garlic peeling, Tetraethyl and methyl lead, thallium (Lunulastreifen), tulip bulbs and flowers, Vanadium, Wet work (e.g. dish-washers, often candida infections),

Narcosis see Coma

Nasal mucosal atrophia, septum perforation, ulceration, atrophic rhinitis

Acute 1. Oxalic acid,
Chronic 1. Antimony, arsenic, Cadmium, chromium (perforation), Phtalic anhydride, Potash ore (perforation),

Nausea and vomiting including Acute gastritis

Acute 1. Acetone, aconite, acrylonitrile, allyl dibromide, aniline, Barium oxide, benzene, benzine, benzyl alcohol, boranes, boron hydrides, butadiene dioxide, Cadmium, carbon monoxide, carbon tetrachloride, chlorine, chloropicrine (trichloronitromethane), cotton dust (mill fever), cyclohexane, Decompression sickness, dichloroacetylene, transdichloroethylene, 2,2--dichloroethyl ether, 2,4-dichlorophenoxyacetic acid, dieldrine, diethyl aniline, diethylene-triamine, 2,2-diethyl-1,3-propanediol, dimethyl aniline, dimethylformamide, dimethylhydantoin-formaldehyde resin, dimethyl sulphoxide, dioxane, diphenylamine, diphenylamine chloroarsine, diphenylcyanoarsine, Ethylamine ketone, ethylene chlorohydrin, ethylene dichloride, ethylene imine, Guaiacol, guanidine hydrochloride, Heat exhaustion, hydrazine, hydrocyanic acid, hydrogen selenide, Inert gases (asphyxia), infra sound, ionising radiation, iron pentacarbonyl, isometheptene, Lead (inorganic), Mercaptans, metal fume fever, methyl bromide, 2-methyl-1-butanol, methyl chloride, methyl dithiocarbamate (together with ethanol ingestion), methylene chloride, methyl propyl carbinol, microwaves, Naphthalene, nickel carbonyl, nicotine, nitroaniline, nitromethane, Organic solvents, organophosphate pesticides, oxalic acid, Parathione (an organophosphate pesticide), perchloroethylene, petroleum naphta, phenol, phosgene, phosphine, phtalic anhydride, polymer fume fever, s-propyl-butyl-ethyl-thiocarbamate (together with ethanol ingestion), propylene oxide, pyridine, Ricinine, Selenium, sodium chloride (e.g. improper use of salt tablets), stibine, styrene, sulphur monoxide, sulphuryl fluoride, Tellurium, tetrachloroethane, tetraethylthiuramdisulphide (TETD), tetramethylthiuramdisulphide (TMTD), (together with ethanol ingestion), thallium, toluene, p-toluene-sulfonyl chloride, trinitromethane, Ultra sound, Vanadium, Water (in connection with NaCl depletion), white spirit, Xylenes,

Chronic 1. Acetonitrile, acrolein, antimony, arsenic, arsine, Benzene, Cresols, cyanides, Dimethylformamide, dinitrobenzene, dioxane, Ethylene dichloride, Extrinsic Allergic Alveolitis (e.g. Farmers' lung), Hydrogen sulphide, Lanthanons ("Rare Earths"), Malt, methanol, methyl chloride, methyl cyanide, Tellurium, tetryl, thiocyanates, Zinc,

    2. 2-Aminothiazole,

Neck rigidity

Chronic 1. Methanol,

Necrosis of skin see Skin dystrophia

Necrosis of teeth see Dental erosions

Nephritis see Kidney diseases

Nephrolithiasis see Stones, renal

Neuralgia esp. n. trigeminus

Chronic 2. Trichloroethylene,

Neurasthenia

Chronic 1. Carbon disulphide, Organic solvents,

Neuritis see Polyneuropathia

Nightmares

Chronic 1. Carbon disulphide,

Nystagmus see also Ataxia and Vertigo

Acute 1. Carbon monoxide, Decompression sickness,
Chronic 1. Ethylene dichloride, ethylene glycol, Mercury, mining (miners'n.),

Obstipatio see Constipation

Obstructive lung disease see Asthma

Ochronosis discolouration of cartilage, tendons and sclerae

Chronic 1. Guaiacol, Phenol,

Odontalgia:

Acute 1. Baro trauma,

3: Toxicity only proven in animal experiments

Oedema, cerebral

Acute 1. Styrene monomer,
  3. 2,2,-dichloroethyl ether,

Oedema, general

Acute 1. Naphthalene, Tellurium, thallium,
Chronic 1. Ankylostomiasis (mining), arsine, Beryllium, Carbon tetrachloride, Phosphine, Tetrachloroethane (even ascites),

Oedema, palpebral, swelling of eyelids

Acute 1. Bromine, PCBs (polychlorinated biphenyls and naphthalenes),
Chronic 1. Acetic acid, arsine,

Oedema pulmonum see Pulmonary oedema

Oliguria see Uraemia

Opistotonus see Convulsions

Optic nerve atrophia see Papilloedema

Optic neuritis see Papilloedema

Osteolysis see Osteomalacia

Osteomalacia including Osteolysis, Osteomyelitis, Osteosclerosis, Milkman syndrome, Skeletal fissures, Spontaneous fractures

Chronic 1. Cadmium, caisson disease, cryolite, Decompression sickness, Fluorides, Mother-of-Pearl (concheolin), Phosporous (yellow), Vibration, vinyl chloride monomer,

Osteosarcoma see cancer of bones

Otitis:

Acute 1. Diving,

Pains, abdominal, including Abdominal tenderness

Acute 1. Acetonitrile, aniline, Cadmium, carbon tetrachloride, caisson disease, Decompression sickness, diethyl aniline, dimethyl aniline, dinitrophenol, dioxane, diphenylamine, Ethylene dioxide, Heat exhaustion, Methyl chloride, Organophosphate pesticides, Parathion (an organophosphate pesticide), phosgene, phosphine, Tellurium, tetrachloroethane, thallium, TOCP, triorthocresyl phosphate,
Chronic 1. Aluminium, arsine, Dimethylformamide, dioxane, Enzymes (proteolytic), Lead (inorganic), Methanol, Tetryl,

Pains of chest see Chest pains

Pains, general

Acute 1. Boranes, Caisson disease, Decompression sickness, Metal fume fever, Polymer fume fever,
Chronic 1. Antimony, Cadmium (itai-itai disease),

Pains of hands, feet and joints

Acute 1. Methylene chloride, Selenium dioxide (esp. fingertips), Thallium, TOCP (triortocresylphosphate),

1: Proven toxicity   2: Suspected toxicity

34

Chronic 1. Allyl chloride, Beryllium, Lead (inorganic), Manganese, Vibration,

Pains of jaw pains on chewing

Acute   1. Dichloroacetylene,

Chronic 1. Mercury (inorganic), mother-of-pearl dust (concheolin),

Pain, precordial see Chest pain

Pallor see Anaemia and Vasospam

Palmar Erythema

Chronic 1. Acrylamide,

Palpitations see Arrythmia

Papilloedema including Optic nerve atrophia, Optic neuritis, Retrobulbar neuritis

Acute   1. Carbon tetrachloride, Dimethyl sulphate, Ethanol, Methyl formate, Organophosphate pesticides,

Chronic 1. Allyl dibromide, aniline, arsenic (organic), Carbon disulphide, carbon tetrachloride, Methanol, methyl bromide, methyl chloride, methyl iodide, Nitrobenzene, Pentachlorophenol, Quinine, Tellurium, thallium, TNT, trinitrotoluene,

   2. Trichloroethylene,

Papilloma see Cancer

Paraesthesia including Hyperaesthesia, Hypoaesthesia

Acute   1. Benzene, Dinitrobenzene, Nitrobenzene, Pyridine methanol, Tellurium, thallium, toluene, Vinyl chloride monomer,

Chronic 1. Acrylamide, arsine, Lead (inorganic),

Paralysis, central including Loss of reflexes, Palsy, Positive Babinski, Ptosis palpebrae

Acute   1. Castrix (2-chloro-4-dimethylamino-6-methyl pyrimidine), Decompression sickness (divers' palsy),

   3. Diphenyl,

Chronic 1. Benzanthrone (corneal and cremaster reflexes), bromates, Cadmium, Methanol (ptosis), methyl chloride (ptosis), Occupational cramps (e.g. writers' cramp), p-Toluene sulfonyl chloride,

Paralysis respiratory see Asphyxia

Parkinson's disease see Extrapyramidal symptoms

Pectus excavatus see Funnel chest

Perspiration see Sweating

Petechiae see Thrombocytopenia

Pharyngitis including Burning throat, Dry mouth, Sore throat, Stomatitis, Xerostomia

3: Toxicity only proven in animal experiments

Acute 1. Aconite, amyl acetate, aniline, Butanol, Cadmium, chromium, colchicine, Dichloro-ethane, dibutylphtalate, diethyl aniline, dimethyl aniline, dimethyl hydantoin formaldehyde resins, dimethyl sulphate, dioxane, diphenylamine, Ethylbenzene, ethylene chloride, ethyl-n-morpholine, formaldehyde, cis-Hexahydrophtalic anhydride, Iso-butylamine, Thomas' slag (basic slag) dust, Zincdimethyldithio carbamate,

Chronic 1. Chromium (ulceration), Mercury (inorganic),

Photophobia see Conjunctivitis

Pleuritis, interlobar

Chronic 1. Silica, amorphous,

Pneumoconiosis see Lung fibrosis

Pneumonitis including Pneumonia

Acute 1. Beryllium, bromine, Cadmium, Ethylene oxide (latent), Hydrogen fluoride, Manganese, mercury, methyl bromide, Sodium hydroxide, sulphuric acid, Thomas' slag (basic slag) dust,

3. Hydrogen selenide,

Chronic 1. Antimony, Dichloroethyl ether, Hydrogen sulphide, Iron pentacarbonyl, Manganese,

Pneumothorax, spontaneous

Chronic 1. Aluminium, Bauxite,

Polycythaemia including Polyglobulia

Chronic 1. Carbon monoxide, cerium, cobalt,

2. Benzene, Manganese, Vanadium,

3. Tetraethyl germanium,

Polyglobulia see Polycythaemia

Polyneuritis see Polyneuropathia

Polyneuropathia motor and sensory see also Paraesthesia

Acute 1. Barium oxide, Compressed air (working in), Ethylene glycol monomethyl ether, Methanol, methyl cellosolve,

Chronic 1. Acrylamide, arsine, Boranes, boron hydrides, Carbon disulphide, cresols, Dinitrophenol, diphenyl, Ethyl iodide, n-Hexane, Lead (inorganic), MBK, methanol (even involving nn. acustici), methyl bromide, methyl n-butyl ketone, Organophosphate pesticides, PCBs, pentachlorophenol, polychlorinated biphenyls and naphthalenes, Tetrachloroethane, tetrachloro ethylene, thallium, TOCP, triortocresyl phosphate, Vibration,

2. Trichloroethylene,

3. 2,3-Dichloro-allyl-diisopropylthiocarbamate, DDT, Lindane, Selenium,

Polyuria

Acute 1. Aconite, Metal fume fever, Polymer fume fever, pyridine,

Chronic 1. Lead (inorganic),

1: Proven toxicity   2: Suspected toxicity

Porphyria, porphyrinuria

Chronic 1. Dimethylformamide, Hexachlorobenzene, Lead (inorganic), Selenium,

Precordial pain see Chest pain

Pressure, raised intraocular

Chronic 1. Ammonia,

Priapismus

Acute 1. Diisocyanates,
Chronic 1. Cyclism (competitive, professional cyclists),

Proteinuria see Albuminuria

Pruritus see Itching

Psychiatric symptoms including Apathia, Behavioural changes, Dementia, Depression, Drunkenness, Ebrietas, Erethismus, Hallucinations, Insomnia, Listlessness, Mania, Melancholia, Psychoneurosis, see also Delirium and Euphoria

Acute 1. Benzene, Carbon disulphide, carbon monoxide, compressed air, (working in), dimethylformamide, dynamite, Metal fume fever, methyl bromide, Nicotine, nitroglycerin, Organic solvents, Perchloroethylene, petroleum naphta, polymer fume fever, pyridine, Styrene monomer, Tetraethyl and methyl lead, thomas' slag (basic slag) dust, toluene, toluidines
Ultrasound, Xylenes,

Chronic 1. Acrylamide, antimony, Boxing (professional), bromides, Carbon disulphide, cyanides, dinitrophenol, dynamite, Lead (inorganic), Manganese, mercury (inorganic), methanol, methyl bromide, methyl chloride, mining (miners' nystagmus), Nitroglycerin, Organic solvents, oxalic acid, Selenium, styrene, Tellurium, toluene, trichloroethylene, Vanadium,

Ptosis palpebrae see Paralysis

Ptyalismus see Salivation

Pulmonary fibrosis see Lung fibrosis

Pulmonary oedema

Acute 1. Acetaldehyde, acrolein, allethrin, ammonia, antimony trichloride, arsine, Benzyl chloride, beryllium, boranes, boron hydrides, bromine, Cadmium, carbon tetrachloride, chlorine, chlorine dioxide, chloropicrine, Deguelin, diazomethane, diisocyanates, diisopropylamine, diphosgene, Ethyl bromide, ethylene chlorohydrin, ethylene dibromide, ethylene dichloride, Hydrofluoric acid, hydrogen selenide, hydrogen sulphide, Isopropylchloroformate, Ketene, Maleic anhydride, methyl bromide, methyl sulphate, Nickel carbonyl, nitrosyl chloride, Organophosphate pesticides, ozone, Phosgene, phosphine, phosporous chlorides, phosporous oxychloride, Selenium dioxide, sulphuric acid, Tetranitromethane, Thomas' slag (basic slag) dust, trichloronitromethane,

3: Toxicity only proven in animal experiments

>   *2.* 1,1-Difluoroethane, Hexamethyldisilane,
>   Methylisocyanate, alpha-Naphthylthiourea,
>   *3.* Allyl glycidyl ether,

Chronic 1. Diazomethane, 2,2'-dichloroethyl ether, dimethyl sulphate,
           Ethylene oxide, Fluorine monoxide, Hydrogen sulphide,
           Nitric acid, nitrous oxides, Polymer fume fever, Sulphur
           dioxide,

Pupil changes including Pupil difference, see also Miosis, Mydriasis

Acute   1. Carbon disulphide, Halogenated hydrocarbons, Methyl
             bromide, methyl chloride, methylene chloride,
             Nitrobenzene, Organophosphate pesticides,

Purging see Diarrhoea

Purpura see Thrombocytopenia

Raucitas see Hoarseness

Raynaud's phenomenon including White fingers

Acute   1. Mercaptans,
Chronic 1. Vibration, vinyl chloride monomer,
Red eye see Conjunctivitis

Reflex disorder see Paralysis and Polyneuropathia

Restlessness

Acute   1. Phosphine, Trimethylene trinitramine,
Respiratory depression see Dyspnoea

Respiratory paralysis see Asphyxia

Retentio urinae see Miction disturbances

Reticulocytosis of erythrocytes

Chronic 1. Aniline, Lead (inorganic),
Retinitis including retinopathy

Chronic 1. Carbon disulphide, laser beams, Iron dust,
             Naphthalene, Quinoline,

Retrobulbar neuritis see Papilloedema

Retrosternal pain see Chest pain

Rhinitis including Coryza, Irritation of nose, Rhinitis vasomotorica,
Rhinorrhoea, Sneezing. See also Nasal mucosal atrophia.

Acute   1. Acetic anhydride, acridine, allylisothiocyanate, ammonia,
             arsenic, Beryllium, bromine, butanol, Calcium cyanamide,
             chlorine, chromium, Dichlorobenzene, 2,2'-dichloroethyl
             ether, dichlorohydrin, diethylaminethyl chloride,
             dimethylaminoethyl chloride, dioxane, diphenyl-
             chloroarsine, diphenylcyanoarsine, Ethyl benzene,
             ethylene dichloride, Formic acid, Hydrozoic acid,
             hydrogen fluoride, hydrogen selenide, hydrogen sulphide,
             Isoprene, MEK, methylethyl ketone, Phosgene, polymer
             fume fever, pyridine, Selenium, styrene, sulphur dioxide,
             sulphur monoxidechloride, TDI, tetrachloroethane,
             Thomas' slag (basic slag) dust, toluene diisocyanate, Zinc
             diethyl-dithio carbamate, zinc dimethyl-dithio carbamate,

Chronic 1. Acacia gum, alfalfa meal, antimony, Cadmium, chloroform, chromium, coffee (dust), cotton (dust), Flour (dust), fluorides, Grain (dust), grain smuts, gum arabic, Hemp (dust), Jute (dust), Linen (dust), Phtalic anhydride, platinum (complex compounds), Saw dust, seeds (dust), Tetryl, thiocyanates, tobacco (dust), Vegetable dust, Wood dust, Xylene,

Rhinorrhoea see Rhinitis

Ringing in ears see Tinnitus

Rose eye see Conjunctivitis

Salivation, excessive s., hypersalivation, ptyalismus

Acute 1. Aconite, acrylonitrile, ammonia, anabasine (mountain tobacco), Cadmium, Organochlorine pesticides, organohosphate pesticides, Parathion, Tellurium, tetrachloroethane, tetrathyl lead,

Chronic 1. Cresols, cyanides, Guaiacol, Manganese, mercury (inorganic), Phenol,

Sarcoidosis (Boeck) see also Lung fibrosis

Chronic 1. Beryllium, Cobalt,

Scleral discolouration see Jaundice and Ochronosis

Sclerodermia

Chronic 1. Vinyl chloride monomer,
       2. Vibration,

Scotoma see Vision disorders

Septum perforation, nasal see Nasal mucosa athrophia

Shivering see also Fever

Acute 1. Boranes, boron hydrides, Cadmium, Manganese, metal fume fever, Polymer fume fever, Zinc oxide, Xylenes,

       2. Zinc stearate,

Shock see Collapse

Shortness of breath see Asthma, Chest pain and Dyspnoea

Sighing respiration see Dyspnoea

Singultus see Hiccup

Skeletal fissures see Osteomalacia

Skin burns see Skin dystrophia

Skin cracking see Skin dystrophia

Skin discolouration see Skin pigmentation

Skin dryness see Skin dystrophia

Skin dystrophia including Acne, Blistering, Burns, Cracking, Dermatitis, Dermatosis, Erythema, Gangrene, Hyperkeratosis, Hypertrophia, Necrosis, Primary irritants

Acute 1. Acetic acid, acetic anhydride, BAL (British Anti Lewisite), benzene sulphonyl chloride, benzine, bromine, n-butanol, Cresol, croton aldehyde, chromic acid, cutting oils, cyanides, Dibutyl maleate, N,N'-di-sec-butyl-para-

---

3: Toxicity only proven in animal experiments

phenylenediamine, 2,6-dichlorobenzonitrile, dichloro-(2-chlorovinyl)-arsine, dichlorophene, 2,4-dichlorophenoxyacetic acid (and compounds), diiso-octyl-acid phosphate, dimethyl-amino-ethyl methacrylate, dimethylcarbamide chloride, dimethylsulfoxide, dinitrophenol, Fiber glass, fluoboric acid, Glass fibers, guaiacol, Hexachloronaphthalene, hexafluoro acetone, hexylene glycol, hydrazine, hydrofluoric acid, hydrogen peroxide, hypochlorites, Iodine, IR-light, isobutylamine, Kerosene, Laser beam, lauroyl peroxide, lewisite, lime, liquid air and gases, Maleic anhydride, MBA (mechlorethamine), methyl bromide, methyl pyrrolidine, methyl toluene sulfonate, methyl vinyl ketone, mineral oil, morpholine, mustard gas, Naphthalene, nitric acid, nitriles, p-nitroso-dimethyl aniline, Oil (mineral), organic solvents, oxalic acid, Peroxides, phenol (gangrene), beta-phenyl-ethylamine, phenyl mercuric hydroxide, phosphorous (yellow), phosphorous acid, phosphorous pentabromide, phosphorous pentachloride, phosphorous pentafluoride, phosphorous pentoxide, phospho-tungstic acid, potassium hydroxide, pyridine perchlorate, pyridine, pyridine methanol, pyromellitic acid, Rotenone (derris), Sabadilla, selenium dioxide, sodium hydroxide, sodium isopropylxanthate, sodium silicate, strong acids, styrene, sulphuric acid, Tantalum, 2,2,4,4-tetramethyl-1,3-cyclobutanediol, thionylchloride, tin (organo-tin compounds), titaniumtetrachloride, toluenediamine, p-toluenesulfonyl chloride, trichloroethylene, triethylene tetramine, trisodium phosphate, Vinyl pyridine, Water glass (Na_2SiO_3), white spirit, Zinc chloride (soldering flux), zinc ethylene bis-(di-thiocarbamate),

Chronic 1. Acetic acid, acetic anhydride, 4-amino-N-diethyl-aniline-sulphate (lichen ruber), amyl laurate, arsenic, asbestos (asbestos corns), benzyl chloride, bromides (inorganic), bromine (brom-acne), n-butanol (esp. around finger nails), Calcium cyanamide, carbon tetrachloride, Cedar wood dust, chromium (chrome holes), coal tar, cold exposure, Dichloroethane, dicycloheptadiene, dimethyl sulphate, Enzymes (proteolytic), ethylenechlorohydrin, ethylene dichloride, Fluorides, formaldehyde, Greenhow's disease, Heat exposure, hydrochloric acid, Nickel, Organic solvents, oxalic acid, Paraffins, PCBs, pitch, platinum, polychlorinated biphenyls and naphthalenes, propane, Resorcinol, Sulphur dioxide, sulphuric acid, Tellurium, tetrachlorobenzodioxine (chloracne), tetra ethyl and methyl lead, trichloroethylene, Vibrations,

Skin gangrene see Skin dystrophia

Skin granuloma including Warts

Chronic 1. Asbestos, asphalt, Beryllium, Coal tar, Mineral oil, Pitch,

Skin healing disorders see Wounds

1: Proven toxicity   2: Suspected toxicity

Skin hypertrophia see Skin dystrophia

Skin necrosis see Skin dystrophia

Skin pigmentation including Depigmentation, Discolouration, Erythema, see also Flush and Leucoderma

Acute 1. Benzene, Heat, IR-light, Nitric acid, Picric acid,

Chronic 1. Aniline, arc welding, arsine, Bromine (yellow discolouration), para-tert-butylphenol, Coal (coal miners' scars), Dinitrobenzene, dinitro-ortocresol, dinitrophenol, Guaiacol, Hydroquinone-mono-benzyl ether, Mercury vapour lamps, metol, PCBs, phenol, polychlorinated biphenyls and naphthalenes, Silver, Tellurium (bluestained finger webs), tetryl, thallium, TNT (only hair), trinitrotoluene (TNT), UV-light,

Skin ulcers see Wounds

Sleep disturbances see also Insomnia and Somnolence

Acute 1. Benzene, Pyridine, Tetraethyl and methyl lead,

Chronic 1. Carbon disulphide, Manganese, mercury (inorganic), Organophosphate pesticides, Toluene,

Sneezing see Rhinitis

Somnolence including Drowsiness, Lethargia, Sleepiness

Acute 1. Acetone, Acetonitrile, Boranes, boron hydrides, butanol, Chlorobenzenes, cyclohexanol, 2,2-Diethyl-1,3-propanediol, dimethylsulphoxide, dioxane, Ethyl alcohol, ethylene chlorohydrin, ethyleneglycol monomethyl ether, ethyl ether, Inert gases (asphyxia), Metal fume fever, methyl bromide, methyl cellosolve, methyl chloride, methyl methacrylate, monochlorobenzene, motion sickness, Organic solvents, Perchloroethylene, phosphine, polymer fume fever, polymethylmethacrylate (vapours), Styrene (and fumes from polystyrene), Tellurium, trichloroethane, trichloroethylene, Ultrasound, Vanadium,

Chronic 1. Acrylamide, Chloroform, Ethylene glycol, Manganese, Tellurium,

Sore throat see Pharyngitis

Speech disorders see Ataxia

Spleen damage unspecified

Acute 1. Hydrogen selenide,

Staggering gait, difficult walk, see also Ataxia

Acute 1. Aniline, Carbon disulphide, carbon monoxide, Dinitrobenzene, Methyl bromide,

Chronic 1. Acrylamide, Methanol, Phosphine, TOCP, triortocresyl phosphate,

Stillbirth see Embryonic development disorders

Stomatitis see Pharyngitis

Stones, renal

Chronic 1. Acetonitrile, Beryllium, Cadmium, Methyl cyanide,

3: Toxicity only proven in animal experiments

Stones, salivary glands

Chronic 1. Beryllium,

Stupor see Coma

Sulphaemoglobinaemia

Chronic 1. Chloropicrine, Sulphonamides, TNT, trichloronitromethane, trinitrotoluene,

Surditas see Deafness

Sweating, excessive s., Hyperhidrosis, Perspiration, Profuse s.

Acute 1. N,N'-Di-sec-butyl-para-phenylenediamine, dinitrocresol, dinitrophenol, Metal fume fever, methyl bromide, Naphthalene, Organophosphate pesticides, Polymer fume fever, TDI, toluene diisocyanate, Vinyl chloride monomer,

Chronic 1. Acrylamide (esp. palmar), Extrinsic Allergic Alveolitis (e.g. Farmers' lung), Malt, manganese, methanol,

Sweating suppression of, Anhidrosis, Ischidrosis

Chronic 1. Tellurium, thallium,

Swelling of eyelids see Oedema, palpebral

Syncope see Collapse

Tachycardia see Arrythmia

Tachypnoea see Dyspnoea

Taste disorders including Ageusia, "Bad taste", Bitter taste, Dysgeusia, Metallic taste

Acute 1. Cadmium, Hydrogen selenide, Mercury, Toluene,

Chronic 1. Antimony, Chromium, Lead (inorganic), Selenium, sulphur dioxide, Tellurium, tetrachloroethane,

Tearing see Conjunctivitis

Teeth see Dental

Tendon discolouration see Ochronosis

Tenesmi

Acute 1. Aconite,

Terminal convulsions see Convulsions

Thirst see also Pharyngitis

Acute 1. Dintrophenol, Metal fume fever, Phosphine, polymer fume fever,

Chronic 1. Mercury (inorganic),

Throat, burning, dry, irritated, sore, see Pharyngitis

Throbbing see Arrythmia

Thrombocytopenia including Blood coagulation defects of other causes, Petechiae

Acute 1. Ethylene glycol monomethyl ether, Ionising radiation, Methyl cellosolve,

Chronic 1. Benzene, Carbon tetrachloride, Dichlorohydrin, Ionising radiation, Lanthanons ("Rare Earths"), Trimethylbenzenes, Xylenes,

1: Proven toxicity   2: Suspected toxicity

2. Dichlorohydrin, dysprosium, Ethylene glycol monomethyl ether, Gadolinium, Holmium, Neodymium, Thiourea,

3. Mesitylene (1,3,5-trimethylbenzene),

Thyroid enlargement including Goiter

Chronic 1. 2-Amino-5-sulfanilylthiazole,

Tinnitus including Ringing in ears

Acute 1. Aniline, Diethyl aniline, dimethyl aniline, diphenylamine, Phenol, Ultrasound,

Tiredness including Asthenia, Fatigue, Langour, Lassitude, Weakness

Acute 1. Acetonitril, 2-amino-pyridine, iso-amyl acetate, aniline, arsine, Benzanthrone, benzene, Carbon disulphide, Dichloroethylene, diethyl aniline, dimethyl aniline, dinitrobenzene, diphenylamine, Ethylene-glycol dinitrate, Guaiacol, Heat exhaustion, hydrogen selenide, Inert gases (asphyxia), Mannitol hexanitrate, metal fume fever, methanol, Nickel carbonyl, nitroaniline, nitrobenzene, Organophosphate pesticides, ozone, Pentachlorophenol, pentaerythritol tetranitrate, PETN, phenol, phosphine, polymer fume fever, Styrene (and fumes from polystyrene), Tellurium, tetraethyl lead, toluene, toluene sulfonyl chloride, toluidines, trichloroethane, trimethyl benzenes, Ultrasound, Vinyl chloride monomer, Xylene,

Chronic 1. Acrylamide, aniline, ankylostomiasis (mining), Beryllium, boranes, boron hydrides, byssinosis, Carbon disulphide, cotton dust, cyanides, Dinitrobenzene, dinitro-ortocresol, dinitrophenol, Extrinsic Allergic Alveolitis (e.g. Farmers' lung), Iodides, Lead (inorganic), Malt, manganese, methyl chloride, methylene chloride, microwaves, Nitrobenzene, Phenyl hydrazine, phosphorous (yellow), phtalic anhydride, Selenium, sodium sulfocyanide, TDI, thallium, toluene, toluene diisocyanate,

2. 2-Aminothiazole, Carbon monoxide, Germanium,

3. Methylcyclopentadienyl manganese tricarbonyl,

Tracheitis see Laryngitis

Tremor see also Extrapyramidal symptoms and Ataxia

Acute 1. Aniline, Boranes, boron hydrides, Dichloroethylene, diethyl aniline, dimethyl aniline, diphenylamine, Ethylglycol monomethyl ether, Heptachlor (an organochlorine pesticide), hydrazine, Methyl bromide, methyl cellosolve, monochlorobenzene, Organophosphate pesticides, Phosphine, Tetraethyl and methyl lead, Vanadium,

3. Ethyl silicate,

Chronic 1. Acrylamide, allyl dibromide, Boranes, boron hydrides, Ethylene dichloride, Manganese, mercury (inorganic), methyl bromide, mining (miners' nystagmus), Occupational cramps (e.g. writers' cramp), Resorcinol, Tetrachloroethane, Vanadium,

3: Toxicity only proven in animal experiments

Trismus

Acute 1. Methyl bromide,

Unconsciousness see Coma

Uraemia including Anuria, Hyperazotaemia, Oliguria

Acute 1. Aconite, Mercury (inorganic), methyl bromide, Pentachlorophenol,

Chronic 1. Boranes, boron hydrides, Carbon tetrachloride, Dinitrophenol, dioxane, Lead (inorganic),

Urine discolouration

Acute 1. Cadmium, Guaiacol, Phenol ("black urine"),

Chronic 1. Aniline, Dinitrobenzene, Guaiacol, Metol, Phenol, Tetrahydronaphthaline (tetraline),

Urine retention see Miction disturbances

Vasoconstriction see Raynaud's phenomenon

Vasodilatation see Flush

Vasospasm see Raynaud's phenomenon

Vertigo including Dizziness, Giddiness, Labyrinthitis, Vestibulitis

Acute 1. Acetic acid, acetone, acetylene, aconite, anabasine (neonicotine), aniline, arsine, Benzine, benzanes, boron hydrides, butanol, Cadmium, calcium cyanamide, cresols, Decompression sickness, dieldrine, diethyl aniline, 2,2-diethyl-1,3-propanediol, dimethyl aniline, dinitrobenzene, dioxane, diphenylamine, Ethylbenzene, ethylenechlorohydrin, ethylenedichloride, ethyleneglycol dinitrate, Guaiacol, Histamine, hydrocyanic acid, hydrogen selenide, hydrogen sulphide, Iron pentacarbonyl, Lindane (gamma-hexachlorocyclohexane), Mannitol hexanitrate, isometheptene, methylacetate, methyl bromide, 2-methyl-1-butanol, methyl chloride, methylene chloride, methyl methacrylate, methyl propyl carbinol, Nickel carbonyl, nitro-benzene, Organophosphate pesticides, ozone, Phenol, phosphine, pyridine methanol, Trichloroethylene, turpentine, Ultrasound, Xylenes,

Chronic 1. Acrylamide, amyl alcohol, aniline, antimony, Boranes, boron hydrides, Chloroform, cyanides, Guaiacol, Gallium fluoride (labyrinthitis), Hydrogen sulphide, Mercury, methanol, mining (miners' nystagmus), monochlorobenzene, Nitriles, nitrobenzene, Phenol, phtalic anhydride, Thiocyanates,

2. Carbon monoxide, Mercaptans,

Vestibular neuritis see Vertigo

Vestibulitis see Vertigo

Vision disorders other than Conjunctivitis and Corneal damage including Blurring, Chalkosis, Dimness, Scotomas, Colour vision defects,

see also Cataract, Diplopia, Miosis, Mydriasis and Pupil changes

1: Proven toxicity   2: Suspected toxicity

44

Acute   1. Anabasine (neonicotine), Carbon monoxide, Hydrogen sulphide, Laser beam, Methanol, methyl acetate, methyl bromide, methyl chloride, methyl iodide, Naphthalene, Organophosphate pesticides, Perchloroethylene, Phenol, Vanadium,

Chronic 1. Boranes, boron hydrides, Carbon disulphide, copper (metallic, chalkosis), Dimethyl sulphate (colour vision), Lead (inorganic), Mercury (inorganic, "mercurialentis"), methanol, methyl mercury (looking-glass vision),

 2. Laser beam, Phosphine,

Vitiligo see Leucoderma and Skin pigmentation

Vomiting see Nausea

Walking difficulties see Ataxia and Staggering gait

Warts see Skin granuloma

Weakness see Tiredness

Weight loss including Emaciation, Cachexia, see also Anorexia

Acute   1. Beryllium, Vanadium,

Chronic 1. Acrylamide, adiponitrile, Benzanthrone, beryllium, bromides (inorganic), Cadmium, Dinitrobenzene, dinitrophenol, Fluorides, Hydrogen sulphide, Iodides, Lead (inoranic), Oxalic acid, Pentachloro-phenol, phenol, Tetramethylene cyanide, toluene, p-toluene sulfonyl chloride,

Wheezing see Asthma

White fingers see Raynaud's phenomenon

Wounds, slow healing

Acute   1. Alkylmethane sulfonoxy derivatives, aluminium, ankylostomiasis (mining), Magnesium,

Wrist drop se Polyneuropathia

Xerostomia see Pharyngitis

X-rays see Radiation, ionising

Yellow line of teeth

Acute   1. Cadmium, chromium,

3: Toxicity only proven in animal experiments

Part II

A GIVEN AGENT:
SIGNS, SYMPTOMS, AND THERAPY

General principles in the therapy of chemical injuries are given here to be used together with the following descriptions of the individual agents. These descriptions are supplied with recommendations – if any – for specific treatment, and some warnings. Our intention is to point out "What to do and what NOT to do in each particular case".

GENERAL PRINCIPLES IN THE TREATMENT OF CHEMICAL INJURIES

The damage is proportional to the concentration and the length of the time the chemical has been in contact with the tissues.

In each individual case it is important to know which chemicals are involved. Even at night the manager in charge must be called in order to ascertain the components of his preparation. If necessary, the police will have to be contacted.

Due to the various possibilities and traditions in treatment in different countries it is not possible to state here where to start treatment.

A. Local damage from caustic agents

Skin:

The remedy of choice is water. Rinse with cold or luke-warm water immediately and continue to do so on the way to hospital. A bucket of water and some rags will do.

Injuries caused by acids or alkalies are controlled with pH-strips (e.g. litmus paper) every $1/2$ hour. If pH differs from 7, continue rinsing. In the case of acids and alkalies DO NOT waste time trying to find neutralizing agents!

In case of contamination with water-insoluble agents, such as organic solvents and oils, wash for 10 minutes with soap and water.

Oil-soluble poisons can be extruded from the skin with vaseline-gauze (to be changed every $1/2$ hour).

Respiratory tract:

a) Inhalation of particles, dusts, aerosols: Rinse with isotonic sodium chloride solution through a tube or bronchoscope (in hospital).

b) Inhalation of irritating gases of fumes: Place the victim in fresh air immediately, give oxygen and/or artifical respiration if necessary.

Beware of latent PULMONARY OEDEMA (see part I)!

Eyes:

Rinse with water – an isotonic solution of sodium chloride if available – for 10-15 minutes. In the case of contamination with alkalies the minimum time is 20 minutes and the eyes should be instilled intermittently with EDTA-eyedrops (to prevent formation of calcium soaps).

B General intoxication.

Absorption through skin:
Immediately rinse with water; take off clothes and wash the skin with water and ordinary soap.

Absorption through airways:
(Narcosis and/or organic damage)
Place the victim in fresh air, in the unconsciousness position, and give oxygen and/or artificial respiration if necessary.
Intoxication with methanol, acetone or halogenated hydrocarbons indicates contacting a centre for renal dialysis.

SIGNS, SYMPTOMS, AND SPECIFIC TREATMENT DUE TO A GIVEN AGENT

Groups 1 and 2 only.

Acute intoxication = A:
Chronic intoxication = C:
Therapy: = Th:

Abrasive dust:
C: Dental erosions
Acacia gum:
A: Conjunctivitis, cough, wheezing, asthma.
C: Rhinitis.
Th: Avoid exposure.
Acetaldehyde:
A: Headache, conjunctivitis, bronchitis, oedema pulmonum, coma.
Acetic acid:
A: Conjunctivitis, headache, vertigo, skin burns.
C: Conjunctivitis, bronchitis, palpebral oedema.
Acetic anhydride:
A: Conjunctivitis, bronchitis, rhinitis, asthma, skin burns.
Th: As acids.
Acetone:
OBS! A potentiator of organic solvents toxicity
esp. carbon tetrachloride
A: Nausea and vomiting, conjunctivitis, foetor ex ore, headache, vertigo, somnolence, coma.
C: Metabolic acidosis, dermatitis (defattening the skin).
Th: Symptomatic, renal dialysis.
Acetone cyanhydrin: (decomposes to hydrogen cyanide and acetone).
Acetonitrile:
A: (Late onset, about 4 hours) chest and abdominal pains, respiratory depression, nausea, vomiting, haematemesis, albuminuria, muscular weakness, renal calculi (oxalate), convulsions, coma, death.
Th: Symptomatic.
Acetyl bromide: (decomposes to hydrobromic acid and acetic acid, when heated to bromine and carbonyl bromide).

Acetylene:

A simple asphyxiant, see Argon.

Acetylene tetrachloride: see Tetrachloroethane.

Acetylhydrazine:

C: Haemolysis.

Acids, esp. strong:

A: Keratitis, skin burns.

C: Dental erosions.

Acetonite, see Aconite.

Aconite: Absorbed through skin, may cause death in from 8 minutes to 4 hours.

A: deafness, salivation, nausea, vomiting, polyuria, diarrhoea, dry mouth, anuria, vertigo, convulsions, tenesmi, mydriasis

Th: Symptomatic, artificial respiration, oxygen.

Acridine:

A: Itching, skin burns, rhinitis.

Acroleine:

A: Conjunctivitis, bronchitis, pulmonary oedema.

C: Conjunctivitis, bronchitis, asthma, headache, nausea, vomiting.

Th: Symptomatic, avoid exposure.

Acrylamide:

A: Conjunctivitis.

C: Palmar hyperhidrosis, somnolence, psychiatric disturbance, weight loss, paraesthesia of limbs, bladder disturbances, vertigo, palmar erythema, lethargy, tremor, gait disturbances (propulsion), conjunctivitis.

Acrylonitrile:

A: Flushing of face, increased salivation, deepened respiration, nausea, vomiting, headache, leucocytosis, mild jaundice.

C: Anaemia, itching, cancer.

Th: Cobalt-EDTA (tetraceminedicobalt).

Adiponitrile:

A: Gastro-intestinal disturbances (unspecified).

C: Weight loss.

Aldehydes:

A: Conjunctivitis, bronchitis.

Aldrin:

A: Convulsions.

Alfalfa meal:

A: Asthma, conjunctivitis, cough, rhinitis.

Alkalies:

A: Keratitis.

C: Dental erosions.

Alkyl methanesulphonoxy derivatives:

C: Slow healing of wounds.

Allethrin:

A: Asthma, pulmonary oedema.

C: Kidney and liver damage.

Allyl alcohols:

A: Conjunctivitis, bronchitis.

Allyl chloride:

A: Conjunctivitis, bronchitis.

C: Pains of hands, feet and joints.

Allyl dibromide:

A: Heart arrythmia, ataxia, conjunctivitis, nausea, vomiting.

C: Optic neuritis, tremor.

Allylene:

A: simple asphyxiant, see Argon.

Allyl iso-thiocyanate:

A: Lachrymation, rhinitis, asthma.

Allylpropyl disulphide:

A: Conjunctivitis, bronchitis.

Aluminium:

A: Bronchitis (carbide and sulphate).

C: Asthma, emphysema, spontaneous pneumothorax, pulmonary fibrosis, dry cough, eosinophilia, chest pains, anorexia, decreased vital capacity, abdominal pains, slow healing of wounds.

Ametocaine (local anaesthetic used by dentists):

C: Nail dystrophia.

Amino-ethyl-ethanolamine:

A: Asthma.

4-Aminofolic acid:

C: Leucopenia.

p-Aminophenol:

C: Asthma, methaemoglobinaemia with cyanosis.

Aminopterin:

C: Anaemia, leucopenia.

2-Aminopyridine:

A: Headache, fatigue, coma.

Aminopyrine:

A: Convulsions.

C: Leucopenia.

p-Aminosalicylic acid:

A: Diarrhoea, anaemia, jaundice.

2-Amino-5-sulphanilylthiazole:

A: Anaemia, haemolysis, haematuria.

C: Goiter.

2-Aminothiazole:

A: Headache, nausea, weakness.

Ammonia:

A: Conjunctivitis, salivation, rhinitis, bronchitis, cyanosis, cough, dyspnoea, corneal ulcers, urinary retention, pulmonary oedema.

C: Raised intraocular pressure (latent).

Th: As for alkalies.

Ammonium bichromate:

C: Asthma.

Amyl acetate:

A: Burning in eyes, lachrymation, headache, dryness of throat, "dopiness", fatigue.

Amyl alcohol:

A: Conjunctivitis, cough, headache.

C: Headache, vertigo.

d-Amyl bromide:

C: Liver disease.

Amyl laurate:

C: Skin dystrophia.

Amyl nitrite:

A: Hypotension, headache.

Anabasine:

A: Salivation, mental confusion, dizziness, disturbed hearing, disturbed vision, unconsciousness, convulsions.

Aniline:

A: Burning throat, chest constriction, nausea, urinary incontinence, dizziness, tinnitus, face flush(bluish grey), tremor, lilac skin, muscular weakness, staggering gait, methaemoglobinaemia; (Severe) abdominal cramps, vomiting, shock, jaundice, coma, convulsions, asphyxia, dyspnoea, haemolysis, death.

C: Basophilia, cyanosis, weakness, fatigue, giddiness, anaemia, ataxia, jaundice, haemoglobinuria, haemolysis, papilloedema, discolouration of urine, reticulocytosis, skin pigmentation.

Th: Remove contaminated clothes. If patient cyanotic (methaemoglobinaemia) give methylthionine 1-2 mg/kg body weight slowly by the intravenous route.
Blood transfusion may be indicated. Symptomatic treatment.

Ankylostomiasis: in mining

C: Anaemia, gastro-intestinal disturbances.

Antimony: see also Stibine

C: Nasal mucosal atrophia, pneumonitis, rhinitis, metallic taste, nausea, vomiting, diarrhoea, psychiatric disturbances, sleepless-ness, fatigue, dizziness, liver disease, leucocytosis, jaundice, muscular pains, gingivitis, anorexia, headache, heart disease (without specification), death.

Th: BAL is indicated.

Antimony trichloride:

A: Pulmonary oedema.

Apoatropine: (atropamine)

A: Conjunctivitis.

Argon: (acts as a simple asphyxiant).

A: Dyspnoea, headache, vertigo, fatigue, nausea, vomiting, somnolence, coma, convulsions, death.

Th: Remove patient to fresh air. Oxygen and artifical respiration if necessary.

Arnica (mountain tobacco):

A: Gastrointestinal disturbances (unspecified), coma.

Aromatic nitro compounds:

C: Cataract,

Arsenic:

A: Gastrointestinal disturbances, rhinitis, laryngitis (hoarseness), bronchitis, conjunctivitis, diarrhoea, vasodilatation, headache, shock, collapse, coma, convulsions, haematemesis, melaena, death.

C: Nausea, vomiting, dermatitis (rain-drop pigmentation) with painful ulcers, nail dystrophia, nasal septum perforation, alopecia, anaemia, anorexia, constipation, convulsions, diarrhoea, glossitis, itching, jaundice, optic neuritis.

Th: Symptomatic, BAL (British Anti Lewisite, dimercaprol).

Arsine:

A: Severe headache, weakness, fainting, vertigo, dyspepsia, jaundice, haemoglobinuria, haemolysis, heart arrythmia, pulmonary oedema, coma, death.

C: Albuminuria, headache, nausea, vomiting, paraesthesia, garlic odour of breath, skin colour change, oedema (face and eyelids), anaemia, basophilic punctuation of erythrocytes, jaundice, epigastric pain.

Th: Symptomatic.

Asbestos:

C: Lung fibrosis, skin granulomata (asbestos corns).

Asphalt:

C: Skin granulomata (warts).

Atropine:

A: Mydriasis.

Bagasse dust: see Extrinsic allergic alveolitis.

BAL (British Anti Lewisite):

A: Conjunctivitis, skin burns.

Barium:

A: Nausea, vomiting, paralysis of legs and arms, cyanosis, dyspnoea.

C: Barytosis, a benign pneumoconiosis.

Barium oxide:

A: Polyneuropathia.

Barotrauma:

A: Odontalgia

54

Bauxite:

C: Emphysema, spontaneous pneumothorax.

Benzanthrone:

C: Anorexia, fatigue, gastritis, hypotonia, impotence, liver disease, reflex disturbances (corneal and cremaster reflexes), tachycardia, weakness, weight loss.

Benzene:

A: Excitement, incoherent speech, facial flush, nausea, vomiting, anorexia, paraesthesia, fatigue (lasting for weeks), erythema of skin, sleep disturbances, coma, death.

C: Epistaxis, thrombocytopenia, aplastic anaemia, leucopenia, abnormal leucocytes, leukaemia, anorexia, haematemesis, leucocytosis, nausea, vomiting, polycythaemia.

Th: Antibiotics, exchange transfusions.

Benzene sulphonyl chloride:

A: Bronchial spasm, Conjunctivitis, skin burns.

C: Hepatitis.

Benzidine:

A: Haemolysis, leucopenia.

Benzine:

A: A simple asphyxiant see Argon.
Bullous skin disease, conjunctivitis, headache, vertigo

C: Impotence.

Benzoyl chloride:

A: Bronchitis.

C: Lung cancer, skin dystrophia.

Benzoyl peroxide:

A: Conjunctivitis, bronchitis.

Benzyl alcohol:

A: Headache, nausea, vomiting, diarrhoea, conjunctivitis.

Benzyl bromide and chloride:

A: Conjunctivitis, oedema pulmonum.

Benzyl dichloride:

A: Conjunctivitis.

Berberine:

A: Gastrointestinal disturbances, hypothermia, death.

Beryllium:

A: Conjunctivitis, cough, retrosternal pain, haemoptysis, chemical pneumonitis, dyspnoea, cyanosis, anorexia, pulmonary oedema, epistaxis, rhinitis, weight loss, death.

C: Chest pain, cough, joint pains, emphysema, hypercalcuria (without hypercalcaemia), skin granulomata, anorexia, oedema, weight loss, renal stones, kidney injury, salivary gland stones, weakness, dyspnoea, liver disease, lung fibrosis (simulating sarcoidosis).

Th: Steroids could be tried.

Bicycloheptadienedibromide:

C: Asthma, injury to blood-forming organs, death.

Bismuth:

C: Gingivitis.

Boranes: see Boron hydrides

Bordeaux mixture: (vineyard sprayers):

C: Liver disease.

Boron hydrides:

A: Vertigo, muscle spasms, heart arrythmia, somnolence, nausea, euphoria, bilirubinaemia, kidney damage (tubuli), chest pain, dyspnoea, hiccup, tremor, coma, convulsions, cough, fever, jaundice, general pains, shivering.

C: Fatigue, vertigo, muscle spasms, bronchitis, polyneuropathia, leucocytosis, liver disease, vision disturbances, headache.

Prevention: Silica gel-containing masks.

Boxing (professional):

C: Cauliflower ears, dementia, boxers' traumatic encephalopathia, punch-drunkenness

bis-1,2-Bromacetoxy-2-butene:

A: Conjunctivitis.

Bromates:

C: Methaemoglobinaemia, paralysis.

Bromides: inorganic

C: Emaciation, skin rashes (esp. of face) "bromoderma", dental erosions.

Bromine:

A: Conjunctivitis, rhinitis, skin burns, bronchitis, dyspnoea, pneumonia, pulmonary oedema, chest pain, palpebral oedema.

C: Skin pigmentation, skin dystrophia "bromacne".

Th: Fresh air, oxygen. Observation for latent pulmonary oedema. Eyes: liquid paraffin and anaesthetic drops.

Bromochloromethane:

A: Conjunctivitis, liver disease, death.

Bromoform:

A: lachrymation, death.

C: Liver damage.

Th: Fresh air, oxygen if necessary.

Butadieneoxide:

A: Conjunctivitis, cough, dyspnoea, headache, hiccup, nausea, vomiting.

Butane: a simple asphyxiant, see Argon.

Butanol:

A. Somnolence, vertigo, conjunctivitis, keratitis, pharyngitis, rhinitis, skin burns, dermatitis.

C: Conjunctivitis, nail dystrophia.

56

Butyl acetate:

A.   Conjunctivitis, bronchitis.

alpha-Butylene:

A simple asphyxiant, see Argon

Butyl glycol:

A: Conjunctivitis, bronchitis.

Butyl nitrite:

A: Hypotension, headache, palpitations, weakness.

para-tert-Butyl phenol:

C: Nail dystrophia.

p-tert-Butyl- toluene.

A: Bronchitis, CNS-depression.

C: Kidney and liver diseases.

Butyraldoxime:

A: Alcohol intolerance, antabus effect, cyanosis.

Byssinosis: see also Mill fever. Dust from cotton, flex and hemp.

A: Symtoms during working day. Chest tightness, cough, dyspnoea, fatigue.

Cacodylic acid:

C: Foetor ex ore.

Cadmium:

A: Inhalation, latent interval of some hours. Cadmium intoxication should be suspected if fever and chest pain persist more than 24 hours in a case of metal fume fever.

Bronchitis, cough, dyspnoea, chest pain, collapse, diarrhoea, fever, chills, headache, coma fatal pulmonary oedema or pneumonitis.

C: Yellow line on teeth, loss of weight, dyspnoea, cough, emphysema (atrophic), kidney disease, albuminuria, raised ESR, rhinitis atrophica, anosmia, amino-aciduria, osteomalacia (milkman fractures), anaemia (iron deficiency type), hypercalcaemia, constipation, diarrhoea, gingivitis, insomnia, hypertension.

Th: Symptomatic. BAL dangerous, should NOT be used!

Caisson disease: see Decompression sickness.

Calcium cyanamide:

A: In connection with ethanol ingestion an antabus reaction may develop: alcohol intolerance, cyanosis, dyspnoea, skin flush, headache, hypotension.

Calcium iodobehenate:

A: Castro-intestinal disturbances.

Calcium oxide:

A: A corrosive, irritating to skin, eyes and mucous membranes,

Th: As for alkalies.

Carbamates:

C: Leukaemia.

Carbon (in the form of soot or graphite):

A: Blepharitis, conjunctivitis, epithelial hyperplasia of cornea, irritation of mucous membranes.

Carbon dioxide:

A: Heart arrythmia, dyspnoea. Acts as a simple asphyxiant, see Argon.

Carbon disulphide:

A: Headache (frontal), drunkenness, hallucinations, pupil changes, staggering gait, muscular weakness, precordial pain, ataxia, conjunctivitis, convulsions, delirium, acute mania, gastro-intestinal disturbances, coma, death.

C: Fatigue, headache, gastro-intestinal disturbances, extrapyramidal symptoms, chronic dementia, polyneuropathia (sensor and motor), somnolence, optic neuritis, auditory disturbances, hypertension, albuminuria, amenorrhoea, anaemia, anorexia, hypercholesterolaemia, euphoria, heart disease (without specification), impotence, nightmares, retinopathy.

Carbon monoxide:

A: Headache, mental confusion, nausea, heart arrythmia, impairment of vision, vomiting, asphyxia, unconsciousness, nystagmus, hypertension, cherry-red face, acidosis (metabolic), staggering gait, death.

C: Polycythaemia, fatigue, vertigo, headache, impotence, insomnia, glucosuria, primary myonecrosis.

Th: Fresh air, oxygen (hyperbar if possible), intravenous sodium hydrocarbonate drip.

Carbon tetrachloride:

A: Headache, diarrhoea, nausea, vomiting, abdominal tenderness (left loin), oliguria, haematuria, narcosis, miction disturbances, pulmonary oedema, death.

C: Leucopenia, general oedema, thrombocytopenia, haematemesis, haemoglobinuria, jaundice, dermatitis, retrobulbar neuritis, kidney and liver necrosis, albuminuria, anaemia, conjunctivitis, epistaxis.

Th: Symptomatic.

Castix (2-chloro-4-dimethyl-amino-6-methyl-pyrimidine):

A: Paralysis.

Cedar wood dust:

A: Conjunctivitis, intense lachrymation.

C: Iridocyclitis, keratitis, dermatitis.

Cerium:

C: Polycythaemia.

Chlorates:

C: Methaemoglobinaemia.

Chlorine:

A: Cough, nausea, vomiting, rhinitis, oedema pulmonum, death. (See also Bromine.)

Chlorine dioxide:

A: Bronchitis, pulmonary oedema.

Chloroacetophenone:

A: A lachrymatory gas (military).

Chloroacetylchloride:

A: A lachrymatory gas (military).

Chlorobenzenes:

A: Somnolence, loss of consciousness, twitching of extremities, red discolouring of urine, dyspnoea, haemoglobinuria.

C: Kidney and liver disease.

1-Chloro-1,1-difluoroethane:

A simple asphyxiant, see Argon.

2-Chloro-4-dimethylamino-6-methyl-pyrimidine:

A: Convulsions

Chloro-fluoro-methane:

A simple asphyxiant, see Argon.

Chloroform:

A: Conjunctivitis, coma.

C: Headache, kidney disease, liver disease, rhinitis, somnolence, vertigo.

Th: Fresh air, oxygen if necessary.

Chloro-nitro benzene:

C: Methaemoglobinaemia, cyanosis.

Chloropicrin:

A: Lachrymation, nausea, vomiting, bronchitis, pulmonary oedema.

C: Sulphaemoglobinaemia.

Chloroprene: (monomer)

A: Conjunctivitis

C: Alopecia (temporary), conjunctivitis, nail dystrophia.

Chlorosulphonic acid:

A: Conjunctivitis, coma.

Chlorotoluidines:

C: Cyanosis, tachycardia, haematuria, albuminuria.

Chromium:

A: Asthma, pharyngitis, rhinitis, skin ulcers.

C: Nasal septum perforation "chrome holes", "chromium enteropathia", diarrhoea, asthma, keratitis, yellow line on teeth, taste disorders, anosmia.

Coal:

C: Skin pigmentation (in scars), lung fibrosis.

Coal tar:

A: Conjunctivitis.

C: Conjunctivitis, skin dystrophia, skin granulomata.

Cobalt (hard metal disease):

A: Chest pain, conjunctivitis, cough, asthma-like symptoms.

C: Polycythaemia, dermatitis (''carboloy itch''), lung fibrosis (after only a few years exposure), bronchitis, cataract, cough, crepitations of lungs, dyspnoea.

Coffee:

C: Amblyopia, hypertension, rhinitis.

Colchicine:

A: Conjunctivitis, pharyngitis.

Cold exposure:

C: Skin dystrophia (perniosis, white spots).

Compressed air, working in:

A: Polyneuropathia, mental confusion.

Copper (metallic):

A: Keratitis.

C: Vision disturbances.

Copper compounds:

A: Haemolysis, metal fume fever, atrophic rhinitis.

Cotarnine chloride:

A: Asphyxia, death.

Cotton dust: see Byssinosis and Mill fever.

Cramps, occupational:

C: (E.g. writers' cramp, telegraphists' c., cotton twisters' c.), spastic, tremulous, neuralgic and paralytic types.

Cresol: (cresylic acid = a mixture of all three isomeres)
Symptoms like phenol but less severe.

Croton aldehyde:

A: Lachrymation, dermatitis.

Cryolite:

C: Anaemia, bone sclerosis, dental erosions, gastrointestinal disturbances, lung fibrosis, osteoclastic metastases (simulating).

Cutting oils:

C: Dermatitis.

Cyan:

A: Death.

Cyanamide:

A: Dyspnoea, skin flush, hypotension.

Cyanides:

A: Dermatitis ''cyanide rash'', collapse, itching.

C: Nausea, vomiting, anorexia, headache, weakness, ataxia, dizziness, conjunctivitis, anosmia, laryngitis, salivation, psychosis.

Th: See Hydrogen cyanide.

Cyanogen bromide and chloride:

A: Bronchitis, conjunctivitis, death.

Cyclohexamine:

A: Convulsions.

Cyclohexane:

A: Conjunctivitis, nausea, vomiting, coma.

Cyclohexanol:

A: Ataxia, headache, somnolence, coma.

Cyclohexanone:

A: Bronchitis, narcosis, asphyxia.

Cyclopentane:

A: Coma.

Cyclopropane:

A: Coma.

Cyclophosphamide:

C: Alopecia, leucopenia.

Cyclotetramethylene oxide:

A: Bronchitis, conjunctivitis.

DDT:

C: Anaemia.

Decaborane: see Boron hydrides.

Decompression sickness (Caisson disease):

A: Paralysis (divers' palsy), subcutaneous emphysema, abdominal pains, general pains, itching, dyspnoea, retrosternal pain, cyanosis, shock, collapse, nausea, vomiting, vertigo, nystagmus, staggering gait, skin flush.

C: Aseptic bone necrosis.

Th: Recompression.

Deguelin:

A: Pulmonary oedema.

Diacetone alcohol:

A: Conjunctivitis.

C: Blood disorders (without specification).

Diacetylene:

A simple asphyxiant, see Argon.

4,4-Diamino-diphenyl methane:

A: Liver injury. ("Epping jaundice")

Dianisidine see Benzidine.

Diazomethane:

A: Bronchitis, cough, pulmonary oedema.

C: Asthma, cough, pulmonary oedema.

Dibenzyl-chloroethyl amine:

C: Leucopenia.

Diborane: see Boron hydrides.

Dibromoethylether:

A: Conjunctivitis.

Dibutylmaleate:

A: Dermatitis.

N,N'-Di-sec-butyl-para-phenylenediamine:

A: Skin burns, sweating, flushing, bradycardia, dyspnoea.

Dibutyl phtalate:

A: Albuminuria, bronchitis, conjunctivitis, headache, pharyngitis.

Dichloroacetylene: (can be formed by thermal decomposition from trichloroethylene)

A: Nausea, vomiting, intensive pains of jaw.

2,6-Dichloro-benzonitrile:

A: Dermatitis.

Dichlorobenzene:

A: Rhinitis, conjunctivitis.

C: Cataract, leukaemia.

Dichlorobenzidine see Benzidine

Dichloro-(2-chlorovinyl)-arsine:

A: Skin dystrophia, death.

Dichloro-diethylsulphide:

A: Leucopenia, lymphadenitis.

Dichloroethane:

A: Conjunctivitis, pharyngitis, rhinitis.

C: Skin cracking, corneal oedema and opacity.

Dichloroethylene:

A: Nausea, vomiting, weakness, tremor, cramps, bronchitis, conjunctivitis.

2,2'-Dichloroethyl ether:

A: Conjunctivitis, rhinitis, bronchitis, nausea, vomiting.

C: Pneumonitis, asthma, emphysema, pulmonary oedema.

Th: Symptomatic.

Dichlorohydrin:

A: Bronchitis, conjunctivitis, rhinitis.

C: Thrombocytopenia.

Dichloromethane:

A: Conjunctivitis, headache.

Dichloromethylarsine:

A: Death.

alpha, beta-Dichloromethyl-ethyl-ketone:

A: Conjunctivitis.

2,3-Dichloro-1,4-naphtoquinone:

A: Conjunctivitis.

Dichlorophene:

A: Skin dystrophia.

2,4-Dichlorophenoxyacetic acid:

C: Kidney injury.

Dichloropropane:
A: Conjunctivitis.
C: Kidney and liver disease.
Dichlorotetrafluoroethane:
A simple asphyxiant, see Argon.

Dicyclo-heptadiene:
C: Skin dystrophia.
Dicyclo-heptadiene dibromide:
C: Anorexia, leucopenia.
Diethyl-amino-ethyl-chloride:
A: Mydriasis, rhinitis.
Di-ethyl-amino-methyl chloride:
A: Mydriasis, rhinitis.
Diethyl aniline: see Aniline.
Diethylene-diamine:
C: Asthma.
Diethylenetriamine:
A: Bronchitis, nausea, vomiting.
C: Asthma.

2,2-Diethyl-1,3-propane diol:
A: Drowsiness, vertigo, nausea, vomiting.
N,N-Diethyl-m-toluamide:
A: Irritating to eyes and mucous membranes.
1,1-Difluoroethane:
A: Coma, pulmonary oedema.
Di-fluoromethane:
A: Bronchitis.

Diisocyanates:
A: Jaundice, liver injury, priapismus, pulmonary oedema.
Di-iso-octyl acid phosphate:
A: Skin dystrophia.
Di-iso-propyl amine:
A: Pulmonary oedema.
Dimethyl-amino-ethyl-methacrylate:
A: Conjunctivitis, skin dystrophia.

N,N-Dimethyl aniline: see Aniline.
Dimethyl carbamide chloride:
A: Conjunctivitis, skin dystrophia.
Dimethyl ether:
A: Coma.
Dimethyl formamide:
A: Conjunctivitis, gastritis, nausea, vomiting, psychiatric disturbances.

C: Porphyria, abdominal pains, hypertension, leucocytosis, liver disease, vomiting.

Dimethyl-hydantoin-formaldehyde resin:

A: Conjunctivitis, sore throat, nausea, vomiting.

C: Abdominal pains.

Dimethylnitroamine:

C: Liver necrosis.

2,3-Dimethylpentanol:

A: Conjunctivitis.

Dimethyl phosphorochloride-thionate (DMPCT):

A: Keratitis

Dimethyl sulphate:

A: Conjunctivitis, pharyngitis, laryngitis, bronchitis, asthma, analgesia, cyanosis.
(Acute latent) pulmonary oedema, leucocytosis, liver injury, cough, kidney injury, heart arrythmia, subcutaneous emphysema, papilloedema, delirium, death.

C: (Delay of several weeks) kidney and liver damage, skin dystrophia, pulmonary oedema, disturbed colour vision.

Dimethyl sulphoxide: (skin absorption)

A: Dermatitis, nausea, vomiting, chills, cramps, lethargy, itching.

Dinitrobenzene: (skin absorption)

A: Headache, vertigo, fatigue, paraesthesia, staggering gait, bluish-grey cyanosis, dyspnoea, coma, death.

C: Methaemoglobinaemia, loss of weight, discolouration of urine, leucopenia, kidney disease, jaundice, fatigue, weakness, headache, liver disease, skin pigmentation, nausea, vomiting, fever, cyanosis, anaemia, deafness.

Dinitroglycol:

A: Hypotension.

C: Arrythmia.

Dinitro-o-cresol: see Dinitrophenol.

Dinitrophenol:

A: Dermatitis, fever, diarrhoea, dyspnoea, anorexia, kidney injury, mydriasis, abdominal pains, sweating, thirst, death.

C: Kidney and liver damages, acidosis (metabolic), cataract, chest pain, cyanosis, diarrhoea, fever, headache, leucopenia, poly-neuropathia, psychiatric disturbances, loss of weight, skin pigmentation, fatigue, uraemia.

Dinitrotoluene:

C: Anaemia, methaemoglobinaemia, cyanosis, liver damage.

Dioxane:

A: Pharyngitis, leucocytosis, nausea, vomiting, abdominal pains, gastro-intestinal disturbances, haemoglobinaemia, kidney injury, anorexia, bronchitis, cough, rhinitis, conjunctivitis, headache, drowsiness, dizziness, coma, death.

C: Nausea, vomiting, abdominal pains, lumbar pains, abdominal and lumbar tenderness, hepatomegalia (without jaundice), albuminuria, anaemia, anorexia, anuria, uraemia, kidney disease, death.

Diphenyl:

C: Liver disease, polyneuropathia.

Diphenyl amine: see Aniline.

Diphenyl-amino-chloro-arsine:

A: Nausea, vomiting.

Diphenylchloroarsine:

A: Headache, nausea, vomiting, rhinitis.

Diphenylcyanoarsine:

A: Conjunctivitis, cold-like symptoms, nausea, vomiting.

Diphenyl ketene:

A: Coma.

Diphenylmethane-4,4-diisocyanate: see MDI

Disphosgene:

A: Pulmonary oedema.

Diving see also Decompression sickness:

A: Otitis

Dynamite:

A: Headache, psychiatric disturbances.

C: Methaemoglobinaemia, psychiatric disturbances.

Dysprosium:

C: Thrombocytopenia.

Electric shock:

A: Heart arrythmia, cataract, leucocytosis, vertebral fractures, death.

C: Myoglobinaemia, kidney disease.

Enzymes, proteolytic:

C: Rhinitis, skin dystrophia, skin ulcers (esp. finger tips), epistaxis, conjunctivitis, glossitis, asthma, retrosternal pain, headache, abdominal pain, lung fibrosis.

Epichlorohydrin:

A: Respiratory paralysis, death.

C: Conjunctivitis, bronchitis, kidney damage.

Epoxi compounds (epoxides):

A: Conjunctivitis.

C: Conjunctivitis, nail dystrophia.

Ethane:

A simple asphyxiant, see Argon.

Ethyl acetate:

A: Conjunctivitis, bronchitis, coma.

C: Anaemia, leucocytosis.

Ethyl alcohol:

A: Conjunctivitis, drowsiness, bronchitis, coma.

C: Optic neuritis, liver disease.

Ethyl amyl ketone:

A: Headache, nausea, conjunctivitis, bronchitis, vomiting.

Ethyl benzene:

A: Conjunctivitis, rhinitis, constriction of chest, pharyngitis, vertigo.

Ethyl bromide:

A: Bronchitis, pulmonary oedema, coma.

C: Kidney and liver damage.

Ethyl carbamate (urethane):

C: Leucopenia.

Ethyl chloride:

A: Narcosis.

Ethylene:

A simple asphyxiant, see Argon.

Ethylene bromide:

A: Bronchitis.

C: Kidney injury.

Ethylene chloride:

A: Pharyngitis.

Ethylene chlorohydrin: (skin absorption, even fatal)

A: Conjunctivitis, sleepiness, drowsiness, headache, myopathia, giddiness, nausea, vomiting, death.

C: Dyspnoea, headache, stupor, skin dystrophia, cyanosis, precordial pain, pulmonary oedema, albuminuria, kidney disease.

Ethylene diamine:

A: Conjunctivitis.

Ethylene dibromide:

A: Conjunctivitis, keratitis, liver injury, pulmonary oedema.

C: Kidney injury.

Ethylene dichloride:

A: Conjunctivitis, keratitis, rhinitis, asphyxia, dyspnoea, narcosis, dizziness, nausea, vomiting, cyanosis, tachycardia, leucocytosis, pulmonary oedema.

C: Dermatitis, anorexia, nausea, vomiting, tremor, nystagmus, kidney injury, leucocytosis, hypoglucaemia, hepato-renal syndrome, delirium, gastro-instestinal disturbances, jaundice.

Ethylene dioxide:

A: Abdominal pains.

Ethylene glycol:

A: Anaemia.

C: Anorexia, nystagmus, somnolence, coma.

Ethylene glycol dinitrate:

A: Vertigo, alcohol intolerance, headache, hypotension, fatigue.

C: Anorexia, death.

Ethylene glycol monomethyl ether (methyl cellosolve):

A: Leucocytosis, tremor, multiple neuritis, somnolence.

C: Thrombocytopenia.

Ethylene imine:

C: Nausea, vomiting, "severe human eye injury".

Ethylene oxide:

A: Cough, dyspnoea, headache, pneumonia (latent), bronchitis, conjunctivitis.

C: Asthma, pulmonary oedema, skin burns.

Ethyl ether:

A: Somnolence, stupor, death from respiratory failure.

C: Anorexia.

Ethyl fluoride:

A: Coma.

Ethyl formate:

A: Conjunctivitis.

Ethyl glycol acetate:

A: Conjunctivitis.

Ethyl iodine:

C: Polyneuropathia.

Ethyl-n-morpholine:

A: Bronchitis, conjunctivitis, pharyngitis.

Ethyl nitrite:

A: Hypotension, methaemoglobinaemia, narcosis.

Ethyl silicate:

A: Conjunctivitis, bronchitis.

Extrinsic allergic alveolitis:

Bagassosis, farmers' lung, mushroom workers' disease, malt workers' dis., maple bark strippers' dis., suberosis, bird breeders' (fanciers') dis., aircondition contamination, sequoiosis, fish meal, furriers' dis., coffee workers' dis., Swiss cheese washers' dis., proteolytic enzyme in laundering detergents.

A: Fever, influenza like symptoms, chills, cough.

C: (Latency of 4-12 hours) nausea, vomiting, fever, cough, headache, raised ESR, haemoptysis, excessive sweating, fatigue, asthma, chest pain, cyanosis, lung fibrosis, coeliac disease (late complication).

Ferrosilicon: (may decompose into arsine and phosphine (q.v.))

Fiber glass:

A: Skin dystrophia.

Flour dust:

C: Dental erosions, Rhinitis.

Fluoroboric acid:

A: Skin dystrophia.

Fluorides:

A: Due to hydrogen fluoride (q.v.).

C: "Fluorosis". Osteosclerosis, osteomalacia, may simulate osteoclastic metastases, "mottled teeth", anorexia, weight loss, anaemia, bronchitis, rhinitis, skin dystrophia, asthma, emphysema, interstitial fibrosis of lungs.

Fluorine:

A: Bronchitis, gastro-intestinal disturbances.

Fluorine monoxide:

C: Pulmonary oedema.

Fluoroacetic acid:

A: Heart arrythmia, convulsions.

Fluoroform:

A: Bronchitis, coma.

Fluorotrichloromethane:

A: Bronchitis.

Formaldehyde:

A: Bronchitis, chest pain, conjunctivitis, cough, pharyngitis.

C: Bronchitis, nail dystrophia, skin dystrophia.

Formic acid:

A: Conjunctivitis, rhinitis.

Furfural:

A: Bronchitis, conjunctivitis.

Gadolinium:

C: Delayed blood clotting.

Gallium fluoride:

C: Labyrinthitis.

Gasoline a simple asphyxiant, see Argon.

A: Conjunctivitis.

Germanium hydride:

A: Haemolysis, death.

Glass fiber: see Fiber glass.

Glycidaldehyde:

A: Bronchitis, miosis.

Glycol: see Ethylene glycol.

Glyodine:

A: Keratitis.

Gold:

C: Conjunctivitis.

Grain dust:

C: Rhinitis.

Grain smuts:

C: Asthma, rhinitis.

Graphite:

A: A nuisance dust.

C: Lung fibrosis.

Grease gun injury:

A: Emphysema, subcutaneous.

Guaiacol: see Phenol.

Guanidine hydrochloride:

A: Nausea, vomiting, diarrhoea.

Gum arabic: see Acacia gum.

Hard metal disease:

    Type I:

A: Chest tightness, cough, asthma.

C: Diffuse interstitial fibrosis of lung.

    Type II:
    Rapid onset of cough, dyspnoea on exertion,
    expectoration, crepitations of lung bases.

Heat: See Infra red light.

Heat exhaustion: (heat load)

A: Nausea, vomiting, abdominal pains, fatigue.

Th: Cooling, fluids, if available potassium per os.

Helium:

A simple asphyxiant, see Argon.

Helvellic acid:

A: Haemolysis, keratitis.

Hemp:

C: Asthma, rhinitis.

2-Heptadecyl-imidazoline:

A: Bronchitis, conjunctivitis.

Heptane:

A: Bronchitis, coma.

Heptylene:

A simple asphyxiant, see Argon.

Hexachlorobenzene:

C: Cutaneous porphyria.

Hexachlorocyclohexane: see Lindane.

Hexachloronaphthalene: (skin absorption)

A: Acneiform eruptions, liver damage.

Hexafluoroacetone:

A: Conjunctivitis, dermatitis.

Hexafluoroethane:

A simple asphyxiant, see Argon.

cis-Hexahydrophtalic anhydride:

A: Conjunctivitis, keratitis, pharyngitis, bronchitis.

Hexamethyldisilane:

C: Alopecia, pulmonary oedema.

Hexamethyl-para-rosaniline:

C: Epistaxis.

n-Hexane:

C: Polyneuropathia.

Hexylene glycol:

A: Bronchitis, conjunctivitis, dermatitis.

Histamine:

A: Flush followed by pallor, dizziness, fainting, headache, tachycardia, hypotension.

Holmium:

C: Anti-coagulant effect.

Hot work see Heat Exhaustion.

Hydrazine: skin absorption

A: Conjunctivitis, dermatitis, nausea, vomiting, bronchitis, convulsions, liver injury, haemolysis, tremor.

C: Kidney and liver disease.

Hydrazoic acid:

A: Conjunctivitis, bronchitis, cough, chills, fever, heart arrythmia, convulsions, headache, skin flush, rhinitis, death.

C: Kidney and liver disease.

Hydrocarbons:

C: Impotence.

Hydrocarbons, halogenated:

A: Pupil changes.

Hydrochloric acid:

A: Bronchitis, gastrointestinal disturbances, laryngeal spasm.

C: Skin burns, dental erosions.

Hydrocyanic acid: see Hydrogen cyanide

Hydrofluoric acid:

A: Nail dystrophia, pulmonary oedema, corrosive to skin, conjunctivitis, convulsions.

Th: Copious rinsing with water seems at the moment to be the only remedy of choice. Injections of calcium-salts are NOT indicated!

Hydrofuramide:

A: Bronchitis, kidney and liver damages.

Hydrogen:

A simple asphyxiant, see Argon.

   OBS! May contain arsine!

70

Hydrogen azide:

A: Conjunctivitis, bronchitis, fever, cough, convulsions, death.

C: Kidney and liver disease.

Hydrogen chloride see hydrochloric acid

Hydrogen cyanide:

A: Asphyxia, ataxia, dyspnoea, chest pain, conjunctivitis, coma, diarrhoea, headache, dizziness, nausea, vomiting, foetor ex ore, death (in minutes).

C: Headache.

Th: Intravenous 300 mg tetracemincobalt immediately, repeat with deterioration. Thereafter 80 ml. of a 15% solution by intravenous route of sodiumthiosulphate.

Hydrogen fluoride (vapours):

A: Bronchitis, conjunctivitis, pneumonia, rhinitis.

Hydrogen selenide: (more toxic than hydrogen sulphide)

A: Conjunctivitis, olfactory fatigue (anosmia), cyanosis, nausea, vomiting, metallic taste, garlicky breath, dizziness, rhinitis, extreme lassitude, dyspnoea, pulmonary oedema.

Th: Vitamin C could be tried; BAL is not indicated.

Hydrogen sulphide:

A: Hyperpnoea, CNS-depression, asphyxia, vertigo, headache, rhinitis, conjunctivitis, disturbed vision, diarrhoea, anosmia, ataxia, delirium, dysuria, euphoria, extrapyramidal symptoms, pulmonary oedema, collapse, death.

C: Conjunctivitis, bronchitis, chest pain, keratitis, headache, dizziness, exhilaration, gastro-intestinal disturbance, cough, diarrhoea, foetor ex ore, nausea, vomiting, vertigo, loss of weight, pulmonary oedema.

Hydroquinone:

A: Keratitis.

C: Pigmentation of conjunctivae.

Hydroquinone monomethyl ether:

C: Leucoderma.

N-Hydroxyethylpyrolidine:

A: Conjunctivitis.

Hydroxylamine:

A: Methaemoglobinaemia.

Hypochlorites:

A: Skin burns.

Hypochlorous acid:

A: Skin burns.

Hyponatraemia: (stokers' cramp)

A: Convulsions.

Inert dusts:

C: Bronchitis.

Inert gases: see Argon.

Infrared light:

A: Cataract, skin flush, erythema of skin.

C: Cataract, skin dystrophia.

Infra sound:

A: Nausea, vomiting.

Iodides:

C: Weakness, anaemia, loss of weight, dental erosions.

Iodine:

A: Bronchitis, chest pain, conjunctivitis, corneal discolouration, cough, skin dystrophia.

IR-light: see Infrared light.

Iron (dust):

A: Conjunctivitis.

C: Siderosis (of tissues where it is deposited). (Metallic dust: retinitis).

Iron nails:

C: Dental erosions (nails held between teeth)

Iron ore (dust):

C: Conjunctivitis, chorioditis.

Iron oxide: see also Metal fume fever

C: Bronchitis.

Iron pentacarbonyl:

A: Dizziness, nausea, vomiting, unconsciousness, (Acute delayed): Chest pains, cough, dyspnoea, fever.

C: Cough, dyspnoea, cyanosis, circulatory collapse, pneumonitis, injury to kidney and liver, death (on 4-11th day after exposure).

Isoamyl acetate:

A: Headache, bronchitis.

Isobornyl thiocyanoacetate:

A: Conjunctivitis, bronchitis.

Isobutane:

A simple asphyxiant, see Argon.

Isobutyl amine:

A: Dermatitis (blistering), headache, dryness of nose and throat.

Iso butylene

A: Simple asphyxiant, see Argon.

Isobutyleneoxide:

A: Conjunctivitis, cough, dyspnoea, headache, hiccup.

Isocyanates:

A: Bronchitis, cough, chest pain.

Isometheptene:

A: Headache, nausea, vomiting, vertigo.

Iso-octane:

A: Coma.

Isophrone:

A: Conjunctivitis.

Isoprene:

A: Conjunctivitis, rhinitis, bronchitis.

Isopropanol: see Isopropyl alcohol,

Isopropylacetate

A: Narcosis.

C: Liver damage.

Iso-propylalcohol:

OBS! A potentiator of organic

solvents toxicity, esp. carbon tetrachloride.

A: Conjunctivitis, foetor ex ore, keratitis.

C: Liver disease.

Iso-propyl-chloroformate:

A: Oedema pulmonum.

Isopropyl ether:

A: Conjunctivitis, bronchitis.

Jute (dust):

C: Rhinitis.

Kerosene:

A: Headache, stupor, dermatitis.

Ketene:

A: Conjunctivitis, pulmonary oedema.

Klordane:

A: Convulsions, death.

C: Anaemia.

Krypton:

A simple asphyxiant, see Argon.

Lanthanum (lanthanons):

C: Nausea, vomiting, delayed blood clotting, haemorrhages, fever, haemolysis, headache, lung fibrosis.

Laser beams:

A: Conjunctivitis, skin dystrophia, disturbed vision, retinal (macular) photocoagualation.

C: Disturbed vision.

Latex, rubber: (contains ammonia (q.v.))

Lauroyl peroxide:

A: Conjunctivitis, skin irritation and burns.

Lead (inorganic):

A: Nausea, vomiting.

C: (Mild intoxication): tiredness, lassitude, abdominal pain, constipation, anaemia, blue line of teeth, albuminuria, hypertension, taste disorders.

(Severe intoxication): wrist drop, ankle drop, muscle tenderness, paraesthesia, encephalopathia, alopecia, amenorrhoea, anorexia, basophilic punctuation of erythrocytes, conjunctivitis, diarrhoea, gingivitis, haemolysis, insomnia, kidney disease, pains of hands, feet and joints, polyuria, porphyrinuria, psychiatric disturbances, reticulocytosis, uraemia, loss of weight.

Lead (organic) see Tetraethyl lead.

Lewisite:

A: Skin dystrophia, death.

Lightning:

A: Cataract.

Lime:

A: Skin burns.

Lindane:

A: Headache, gastro-intestinal disturbances, diarrhoea, convulsions.

C: Aplastic anaemia, bronchitis, conjunctivitis, leucopenia.

Linen dust:

C: Rhinitis.

LPG (Liquefied petroleum gas): see Liquefied hydrocarbon gas.

Liquefied hydrocarbon gas:

A simple asphyxiant, see Argon.

Liquid air and gases:

A: Skin burns.

Lithium:

C: Extrapyramidal symptoms.

Lung fibrosis:

C: Clubbing of fingers, dyspnoea, chest pain, cyanosis, decreased vital capacity.

Maleic anhydride:

A: Keratitis, skin burns, pulmonary oedema.

C: Corneal oedema.

Malt: see Extrinsic allergic alveolitis.

Manganese

A: Fever, shivering, metal fume fever, pneumonia.

C: Tiredness, somnolence, tremor, involuntary movements, uncontrollable laughter, parkinsonism, excessive sweating, hypersalivation, speech disturbances, pneumonitis, psychosis (reversible, other symptoms not), polycythaemia, anaemia, leucopenia, anorexia, emphysema, haemolysis, headache, pains of joints, hands and feet, dental erosions.

Th: Symptomatic; 1-dopa. Neither BAL or EDTA are of any use.

Mannitol hexanitrate:

A: Hypotension, weakness, headache, dizziness.

C: Methaemoglobinaemia, cyanosis.

MBA (mechlorethamine):

A: Skin dystrophia.

MDI (diphenyl-methane-4,4-diisocyanate):

C: Asthma, respiratory disturbances.

Mercaptans:

A: Nausea, headache, cyanosis, Raynaud's phenomenon, vomiting, collapse.

C: Albuminuria, vertigo.

Mercury (inorganic):

A: Fever, kidney injury, pharyngitis, pneumonia, anuria, metallic taste.

C: Alopecia, amnesia, anorexia, ataxia, blue line of teeth, constipation, convulsions, diarrhoea, extrapyramidal symptoms, gastro-intestinal disturbances, gingivitis, headache, impotence, miction disturbances, nystagmus, pains of jaws, psychiatric disturbances, hypersalivation, sleep disturbances, thirst, tremor, vertigo, mercurialentis (eyes).

Th: BAL indicated by the intramuscular route. Further symptomatic therapy, dialysis if necessary.

Mercury (organic): skin absorption

A: (Alkyl mercurials much more toxic than the aryl compounds). Asphyxia, chest pains, cough, dyspnoea, death (methyl m.).

C: Deafness (methyl m.), extrapyramidal symptoms, looking-glass vision.

Mercury vapour lamps: see UV-light.

Mesityl oxide:

A: Keratitis, coma.

Metaldehyde:

A: Conjunctivitis, kidney and liver damage.

C: Kidney disease.

Metal fume fever: (Be, Cd, Cu, Fe, Mg, Mn, Zn)

A: Thirst, headache, profuse sweating, chest pains, fever, dry cough, nausea, vomiting, shivering, fatigue, limb pains, leucocytosis, polyuria, diarrhoea, somnolence, mania, influenza like symptoms. (Recovery after 24 hours; if longer, cadmium should be suspected.)

Methane:

A simple asphyxiant, see Argon.

Methanol:

A: Conjunctivitis, fatigue, arrythmia, dyspnoea, photophobia, foetor ex ore, polyneuropathia, upper abdominal colics.

C: Dizziness, neck rigidity, anorexia, nausea, vomiting, blurring of vision, blindness, palpebral ptosis, coma, metabolic acidosis, deafness, polyneuropathia (involving nn. acustici), abdominal pains, constricted visual fields, diplopia, acute mania, oedema of retina and discs, death.

Th: Ethanol, alkalization.

Methoxychlor (DMDT):

C: Kidney injury.

Methyl acetate:

A: Dyspnoea, palpitations of heart, dizziness, coma, bronchitis, headache, disturbed vision.

Methyl acrylate:

A: Conjunctivitis.

Methyl alcohol: see Methanol.

Methyl bromide:

A: Headache, nausea, vomiting, dimness of vision, euphoria, delirium, staggering of gait, oliguria, mydriasis, trismus, ataxia, bronchitis, conjunctivitis, cyanosis, fever, pneumonia, somnolence, coma, death.

    (Acute latency of 4-48 hours) Tremor, dermatitis with vesication, burns of skin, tremor, vertigo, diplopia, acute mania, pulmonary oedema, convulsions, sweating.

C: Delirium, diplopia, papilloedema, CNS-disorders, tremor, polyneuropathia.

Th: Symptomatic, but continued bed rest and medical observation is mandatory.

2-Methyl-1-butanol:

A: Cough, nausea, vomiting, vertigo, conjunctivitis, bronchitis, giddiness, headache.

C: Deafness, delirium, methaemoglobinaemia.

Methyl butene:

A simple asphyxiant, see Argon.

Methyl-n-butyl ketone:

C: Polyneuropathia.

Methyl cellosolve (ethylene glycol monomethyl ether):

A: Anaemia, polyneuropathia, somnolence.

Methyl chloride:

A: Headache, dizziness, diarrhoea, death, ataxia, coma, euphoria, kidney injury, abdominal pain, pupil changes, fever, albuminuria, nausea, vomiting, drowsiness, blurred vision, accomodation difficulties, delirium at night, tachypnoea.

C: Weakness, anorexia, anaemia, nausea, vomiting, depression, diplopia, ptosis, haematuria, papilloedema, liver disease, haemorrhagia in lungs, meninges and intestinal tracts, headache, kidney disease, leucocytosis, death.

Methyl cyanide:

A: Chest pain, dyspnoea, haematemesis.

C: Coma, convulsions, diarrhoea, nausea, vomiting, renal stones.

Methylcyclohexanone:

C: Kidney and liver disease.

Methyl dithiocarbamate:

A: Collapse, (together with ethanol intoxication) nausea and vomiting.

Methylene chloride:

A: Nausea, vomiting, pupil changes, dizziness, stupor, pain of fingers, keratitis.

C: Fatigue, amnesia, cholesterolaemia, heart disease.

Methylene dianiline:

A: Liver injury.

C: Jaundice.

Methyl ethyl ketone:

A: Bronchitis, conjunctivitis, rhinitis.

Methyl ethyl ketone peroxide:

A: Conjunctivitis.

Methyl ethyl ketoxime:

C: Nail dystrophia.

Methyl formate:

A: Conjunctivitis, optic neuritis.

Methyl glycol:

C: Anaemia.

Methyl iodide:

A: Vision disturbances, narcosis, kidney injury.

C: Papilloedema.

Methyl isobutyl ketone:

A: Conjunctivitis, bronchitis, coma.

Methyl isocyanate:

A: Pulmonary oedema.

Methyl methacrylate:

A: Irritating to mucous membranes, dizziness, drowsiness, loss of consciouness.

Methyl nitrate:

A: Headache, narcosis.

Methyl nitrite:

A: Coma.

Methyl propyl carbinol:

A: Bronchitis, conjunctivitis, cough, headache, deafness, delirium, glucosuria, nausea, vomiting, vertigo, methaemoglobinaemia.

Methylpyridine:

A: Bronchitis.

Methyl pyrrolidine:

A: Skin dystrophia.

o-Methyl silicate:

C: Keratitis.

Methyl sulphoxide: see Dimethyl sulphoxide.

Methyl toluene sulphonate:

A: Skin dystrophia.

Methyl vinyl ketone:

A: Conjunctivitis, skin dystrophia.

Metol:

C: Methaemoglobinaemia, skin pigmentation, urine discolouration.

MIBK: see Methyl iso-butyl ketone.

Mica:

C: Lung fibrosis.

Microwaves:

A: Cataract, nausea, vomiting.

C: Headache, impotence, fatigue, hypertension.

Mill fever:

A: (Cotton dust): headache, cough, fever, nausea, vomiting.

Mineral oil:

A: Skin dystrophia.

C: Skin granulomata.

Mining:

1) Ankylostomiasis.

C: Dyspnoea, general oedema, fatigue, slow healing of wounds.

2) Miners' nystagmus.

C: Blepharospasm, psychoneurosis, nystagmus, vertigo, headache (occipital), head tremor, insomnia.

Monochlorobenzene:

A: Bronchitis, somnolence, tremor, conjunctivitis, cyanosis.

C: Vertigo, headache, coma.

Mono-isopropanol amine (MIPA):

A: Conjunctivitis.

Morpholines:

A: Conjunctivitis, skin dystrophia.

C: Corneal oedema.

Mother-of-pearl dust:

C: Osteomyelitis, osteosclerosis, pains of jaw.

Mustard gas:

A: Leucopenia, lymphadenitis, skin blistering.

Naphthalene:

A: Nausea, vomiting, diaphoresis, haematuria, fever, conjunctivitis, skin dystrophia, general oedema, gastro-intestinal disturbances, convulsions, coma.

C: Liver damage, anaemia, cataract, retinitis, disturbed vision.

alpha-Naphthol: (skin absorption)

A: Keratitis (even injury to lens), kidney damage.

alpha-Naphthyl thiourea:

A: Fever, pulmonary oedema.

C: Leucopenia.

Neodymium:

C: Anti-coagulant effect.

Nickel carbonyl:

A: Haemoptysis, liver injury, fatigue, dyspnoea, vertigo, nausea, vomiting, headache, chest pain, cough, cyanosis, coma.

C: (Latency of 12-36 hours) fever, cough, pulmonary oedema, coma, death.

Th: BAL could be tried, EDTA of no use.

Nickel compounds:

C: Dermatitis "nickel itch", dental discoloration.

Nicotine:

A: Nausea, vomiting, diarrhoea, mental disturbances, convulsions.

Nitric acid:

A: Conjunctivitis, bronchitis, yellow discolouration of skin.

C: Bronchitis, pulmonary oedema.

Nitriles:

A: Skin dystrophia.

C: Bronchitis, vertigo.

Nitrites:

C: Methaemoglobinaemia.

Th: See Aniline.

Nitroaniline: (skin absorption)

A: Headache, nausea, vomiting, weakness, stupor, cyanosis, methaemoglobinaemia.

C: Liver damage.

Nitrobenzene:

A: Dyspnoea, gastro-intestinal disturbances, cyanosis, methaemoglobinaemia, fatigue, vertigo, paraesthesia, miosis, haemolysis.

C: Fatigue, weakness, headache, vertigo, papilloedema, liver disease, anaemia.

Nitrocellulose:

C: Dental erosions (hazard from nitrous oxides).

N-alpha-(1-Nitroethyl)-benzyl-ethylenediamine:

A: Conjunctivitis.

Nitrogen:

A simple asphyxiant, see Argon, Decompression sickness and Liquid air.

Nitrogen mustard:

C: Conjunctivitis.

Nitroglycerin: (skin absorption)

A: Headache, depression, confusion, delirium.

C: Cyanosis, methaemoglobinaemia.
Nitroglycerin together with ethanol ingestion: Dynamite encephalosis (acute mania).

Nitromethane:

A: Anorexia, nausea, vomiting, diarrhoea.

2-Nitropropane:

A: Gastro-intestinal disturbances, kidney and liver damage, methaemoglobinaemia.

n-Nitrosodimethylamine:

A: Skin dystrophia.

Nitrosylchloride:

A: Pulmonary oedema, death.

Nitrous oxides:

A: Heart arrythmia, bronchitis, cough, dyspnoea, cerebral haemorrhage.

C: Insomnia, pulmonary oedema (latent!), pulmonary emphysema.

Th: Symptomatic.

Noble gases: see Argon.

Noise

A: Deafness.

C: Deafness, hypertension.

n-Nonane:

A: Bronchitis.

Octane:

A simple asphyxiant, see Argon.

Oil, mineral: see Mineral oil.

Onions and garlic peeling:

C: Nail dystrophia.

Organic solvents:

A: Coma, conjunctivitis, gastro-intestinal disturbances, headache, skin dystrophia, nausea, vomiting, somnolence, ataxia.

C: Neurasthenia, leucocytosis, skin dystrophia, cataract.

Organochlorine pesticides:

A: Asphyxia, blindness, coma, headache, convulsions, gastro-intestinal disturbances, nausea, vomiting, salivation, tremor, death.

C: Kidney and liver injury.

Th: Calcium gluconate intravenous, phenobarbital against convulsions, further symptomatic therapy.

Organophosphate pesticides:

A: Anorexia, heart arrythmia, vision disturbances, vertigo, asphyxia, ataxia, pulmonary oedema, bronchitis, chest pain, coma, convulsions, cyanosis, diarrhoea, fatigue, gastro-intestinal disturbances, miosis, nausea, salivation, sweating, vomiting, papilloedema, abdominal pains, death.

C: Low cholinesterase level, polyneuropathia, sleep disturbances.

Th: Remove contaminated clothes, rinse with water.
Systemically, atropine 2-4 mg (sic!) by intravenous route,
obidoximchloride 250 mg intravenously or intramuscularly, oxygen
and artificical respiration if necessary.
The rescuer(s) must be kept under observation if unprotected,
has removed contaminated clothes or been giving artificial
respiration mouth-to-mouth.

Osmium tetroxide:

A: Bronchitis, conjunctivitis, keratitis.

C: Asthma, chest pains, headache, conjunctivitis, keratitis.

Oxalic acid:

A: Bronchitis, albuminuria, dermatitis, conjunctivitis, epistaxis,
headache, nausea, vomiting, nasal mucosal atrophia.

C: Loss of weight, irritability, nervousness, chronic cough,
slow healing skin ulcers.

Oxygen, pure (divers, hyperbaric chambers):

A: Euphoria.

Ozone:

A: Headache, vertigo, bronchitis, conjunctivitis, fatigue, chest pains,
hypotension, pulmonary oedema.

C: Asthma, lung fibrosis.

Paraffins:

C: Skin dystrophia.

Paraquat (a herbicide):

A: Anaemia, jaundice, lung fibrosis, death.

C: Liver disease.

Th: Remove clothes, rinse with water (eyes and skin).
If ingested it should be noticed that activated carbon is
ineffective (use Fuller's earth).

PCB's: see Polychlorinated biphenyls and naphthalenes.

Pentachlorophenol:

A: Dyspnoea, fatigue, oliguria, hyperglucaemia.

C: Kidney and liver injury, polyneuropathia, retrobulbar neuritis,
anorexia, loss of weight.

Penta erythritol tetranitrate:

A: Headache, hypotension, fatigue.

Pentamethyl-parafuchsin:

A: Conjunctivitis.

Pentanone:

A: Conjunctivitis, bronchitis, narcosis.

Perchloroethylene (syn. Tetrachloroethylene):

A: Conjunctivitis, bronchitis, nausea, vomiting, drowsiness,
ebrietas, attitude of irresponsibility (severe intoxication),
mental confusion, temporary blurring of vision.

C: Polyneuropathia.

Perchlorylfluoride: (skin absorption)

A: Cyanosis, methaemoglobinaemia.

Perfluoro-iso-butylene: (skin absorption)

A: Cyanosis, methaemoglobinaemia.

Peroxides:

A: Bronchitis, conjunctivitis, skin burns.

Petroleum naphta: (inhalation)

A: Headache, nausea, coma, "haemorages in vital organs", psychiatric disturbances.

C: Diplopia.

Phenol:

A: Muscular weakness, headache, dizziness, black urine, tinnitus, tachypnoea, collapse, convulsions, heart arrythmia, blindness, coma, hypothermia, skin burns and gangrene, death.

C: Loss of weight, anorexia, conjunctivitis, bronchitis, headache, vertigo, diarrhoea, gastro-intestinal disturbances, kidney disease, liver disease, ochronosis, hypersalivation, skin depigmentation, death.

Th: Immediate washing with water (remove clothes), thereafter washing with ethanol or olive oil..

Death may follow in a very short time by only skin absorption.

Phenothiazine:

C: Haemolysis, liver disease.

para-Phenylenediamine:

C: Asthma, fatal liver disease.

beta-Phenyl-ethylamine:

A: Skin dystrophia.

Phenyl ethylene: see Styrene.

Phenyl hydrazine:

C: General weakness, gastro-intestinal disturbances, kidney disease, haemolytic anaemia, liver disease.

Phenyl mercaptan:

C: Headache:

Phenyl mercuric hydroxide:

A: Skin dystrophia.

N-(1-Phenyl-2-nitro-propyl)-piperazine:

A: Conjunctivitis.

Phosgene:

A: Anosmia, conjunctivitis, cough, nausea, vomiting, abdominal pains, rhinitis. (Latent) pulmonary oedema.

C: Asthma, emphysema pulmonum, subcutaneous emphysema, lung abscesses.

Th: Symptomatic. Must be kept under observation for 48 hours in hospital to guard against acute pulmonary oedema.

Hexamethylenetetramine (e.g. Hiprex®) 3 g per os + 20 ml 20% solution intravenously may diminish the risk of latent pulmonary oedema.

Phosphine:

A: Restlessness, fatigue, tremor, drowsiness, bronchitis, thirst, nausea, vomiting, diarrhoea, headache, dizziness, chest oppression, substernal pain, anorexia, dyspnoea, pulmonary oedema, abdominal pain, convulsions, coma, death.

C: Anaemia, bronchitis, gastro-intestinal disturbances, visual disturbances, staggering gait, epistaxis, general oedema.

Th: Symptomatic.

Phosphorous, white:

A: Skin burns, foetor ex ore.

C: Anorexia, jaundice, osteomyelitis "fossy jaw", gastro-intestinal disturbances.

Th: Skin contamination: wash with a solution of copper(II)sulphate.

Phosporous acid:

A: Conjunctivitis, skin burns.

Phosphorous oxychloride:

A: Bronchitis, conjunctivitis, pulmonary oedema.

C: Asthma.

Phosphorous pentabromide:

A: Skin burns.

Phosphorous pentachloride:

A: Bronchitis, conjunctivitis, dyspnoea, haemoptysis, skin dystrophia.

Phosphorous pentafluoride:

A: Conjunctivitis, skin burns.

Phosphorous pentoxide:

A: Bronchitis, conjunctivitis, skin dystrophia.

Phosphorous trichloride:

A: Bronchitis, conjunctivitis, dyspnoea, haemoptysis.

Phosphotungstic acid:

A: Skin dystrophia.

Phtalic anhydride:

A: Nausea, vomiting, cough, asthma bronchiale, headache, hoarseness, bronchitis.

C: Fatigue, vertigo, bronchitis, epistaxis, laryngitis, leucocytosis, nasal mucosa atrophia.

Physical effort, heavy:

A: Myoglobinaemia.

C: Albuminuria.

Picoline:

A: Bronchitis.

Picric acid:

A: Yellow skin pigmentation.

Piperazine:

A: Asthma.

Pitch:

A: Conjunctivitis.

C: Conjunctivitis, skin dystrophia, skin granulomata.

Platinum, complex compounds:

C: Irritation of nose, rhinitis "platinum rhinorrhoea", violent sneeze, chest tightness, dermatitis "platinum urticaria", asthma, cough, bronchitis, cyanosis.

Th: Symptomatic.

Plutonium:

C: Leukaemia, osteosarcoma, pulmonary cancer.

Polychlorinated biphenyls and naphtalenes:

A: Swelling of eyelids, dyspepsia, acute yellow atrophy of liver.

C: Dermatitis "cable rash", chloronaphthalene acne, itching acne, skin hyperpigmentation, jaundice, gastro-intestinal disturbances.

Polymer fume fever:

A: Rhinitis, somnolence, thirst, fatigue, general pains, polyuria, psychiatric disturbances, influenza-like symptoms, leucocytosis, shivering, sweating, chest pain, cough, diarrhoea, fever, headache, muscle pains, nausea, vomiting.

C: Pulmonary oedema (latent).

Th: Symptomatic.

Polymethyl-meth-acrylate fumes:

A: Anorexia, headache, hypotension, somnolence.

Polytetrafluoroethylene (Teflon):

(When heated emits vapours causing Polymer fume fever (q.v.))

Polyvinylchloride fumes:

C: Asthma, "meat wrappers' asthma".

Potash ore:

C: Nasal septum perforation.

Potassium chlorate:

A: Methaemoglobinaemia.

C: Anaemia.

Potassium hydroxide:

A: Conjunctivitis, skin burns.

Potassium perchlorate:

A: Skin dystrophia.

Potassium permanganate:

A: Keratitis.

Pressure, local:

A: Dupuytren's contracture.

Propane:

A: A simple asphyxiant see Argon.

C: Skin dystrophia.

s-Propyl-butylethyl-thiocarbamate:

A: Violent vomiting when accompanied by ethanol ingestion.

Propylene oxide:

A: Headache, nausea, vomiting.

Propylnitrate: (inhalation)

A: Hypotension.

C: Methaemoglobinaemia.

Propyl nitrite:

A: Hypotension.

Pseudocumene:

C: Anaemia, bronchitis.

Pyretrins:

A: Ataxia, collapse, convulsions, diarrhoea, dyspnoea, headache.

Pyridine:

A: Dermatitis, rhinitis, sleep disturbances, CNS-depression,
     gastro-intestinal disturbances, anorexia, conjunctivitis, headache,
     nausea, vomiting, psychiatric disturbances.

C: Diplopia, kidney and liver disease.

3-Pyridine-methanol:

A: Gastro-intestinal disturbances, skin flush, dizziness,
     paraesthesia.

Pyrocatechol:

A: Convulsions.

C: Anaemia.

Pyromellitic acid:

A: Skin dystrophia.

Quartz dust:

C: Lung fibrosis, emphysema, interlobar pleuritis.

Quick lime: see Calcium oxide.

Quinine:

A: Conjunctivitis.

C: Papilloedema.

Quinoline:

C: Retinitis.

Quinone:

A: Pigmented conjunctivae and corneae.

C: Keratitis.

Radiation, heat: see Infra red light.

Radiation, ionizing:

A: Fever, nausea, vomiting, thrombopenia.

C: Anorexia, fever, lymphopenia, thrombopenia, cataract,
     leukaemia, cancer, dental erosions, death.

Raynaud's phenomenon "white fingers":

Pallor, cyanosis precipitated by cold, skin nutritional deficiences.

Resorcinol: (skin absorption)

A: Conjunctivitis, tachycardia, convulsions, death.

C: Dermatitis, enlarged lymph nodes, methaemoglobinaemia, cyanosis, dyspnoea, hypothermia, tremor.

Ricin: (inhalation)

A: Conjunctivitis, haemolysis, diarrhoea, collapse, death.

Ricinine: (inhalation)

A: Nausea, vomiting, dyspnoea, kidney and liver damage, convulsions,coma, death.

Rotenone (Derris, an insecticide):

A: Dermatitis.

Ruthenium tetroxide:

A: Conjunctivitis.

Sabadilla (a botanical insecticide):

A: Dermatitis.

Saw dust:

C: Asthma, conjunctivitis, rhinitis.

Seeds dust:

C: Rhinitis.

Selenium: (compounds and Se-fumes)

A: Nausea, vomiting, garlicky breath, gastro-intestinal disturbances, coryza, lachrymation, anosmia, epistaxis, chest pain, cough.

C: Garlicky breath, taste disorders, gingivitis, liver disease, psychiatric disturbances, fatigue, cataract, dental caries, gastro-intestinal disturbances, headache, porphyrinuria.

Th: Vitamin C could be tried; BAL is NOT indicated.

Selenium dioxide:

A: Pains in finger tips, red discolouring of nails, tenderness of nail beds, dermatitis, pulmonary oedema.

Selenium hydride:

A: Bronchitis.

Silica: see Quartz.

Silver:

C: Pigmentation of conjunctivae and skin.

Sodium aminophenol arsonate:

C: Blindness.

Sodium chloride:

A: Conjunctivitis, nausea, vomiting.

Sodium hydroxide (Caustic soda):

A: Keratitis, pneumonia, skin burns.

Sodium isopropylxanthate:

A: Conjunctivitis, skin dystrophia.

Sodium nitroprusside:

A: Hypotension.

Sodium silicate:

A: Skin dystrophia.

Sodium sulphocyanide:

C: Delirium, diarrhoea, fatigue.

Soman (fluoromethyl pinacolyloxyphosphine oxide):

Liberates hydrogen fluoride.

A: Keratitis, death (15 minutes after skin absorption).

Stibine:

A: Haemolytic anaemia, haemoglobinuria, headache, jaundice, nausea, vomiting.

Strontium hydroxide:

C: Keratitis.

Styrene monomer (even fumes from polystyrene):

A: "Styrene sickness" (different from polymer fume fever): Nausea, vomiting, headache, fatigue and dizziness.

(Further acute symptoms) Conjunctivitis, lachrymation, keratitis, rhinitis, bronchitis, narcosis, dermatitis (skin defattening), oedema cerebri, psychiatric disturbances, convulsions, somnolence, death,

C: Encephalopathia, psychiatric disturbances, toxic hepatitis.

Sugar:

C: Dental erosions.

Sulphonamides:

C: Sulphaemoglobinaemia.

Sulphur:

C: Bronchitis.

Sulphur chloride:

A: Conjunctivitis, rhinitis, bronchitis.

Sulphur dioxide:

A: Conjunctivitis, dyspnoea, rhinitis, bronchitis, cough, coma, death.

C: Anosmia, bronchitis, chest pain, taste disorders, skin dystrophia, conjunctivitis, dental erosions, extrapyramidal symptoms, pulmonary oedema.

Sulphuric acid:

A: Dermatitis, skin burns, skin necrosis, conjunctivitis, bronchitis, chemical pneumonitis, pulmonary oedema.

Sulphur monoxide:

A: Nausea, vomiting.

Sulphur trioxide:

A: Bronchitis.

Sulphuryl chloride:

A: Itching.

C: Bronchitis.

Sulphuryl fluorides:

A: Nausea, vomiting, cramps.

Tabun (a nerve gas):

A: Keratitis.

Tantalum:

A: Skin dystrophia.

Tar dust:

A: Conjunctivitis.

C: Conjunctivitis.

Tartaric acid:

C: Dental erosions.

Tellurium:

A: Salivation, somnolence, abdominal pains, paraesthesia, garlic odour of breath and sweat, general oedema, fatigue, albuminuria, nausea, vomiting, diarrhoea, eosinophilia, leucocytosis.

C: Garlic odour of breath and sweat, blue staining of finger webs, extrapyramidal symptoms, gastro-intestinal symptoms, headache, nausea, vomiting, metallic taste, anorexia, constipation, dry skin (suppression of sweat), somnolence, papilloedema, depression, cataract.

Tellurium hexafluoride:

A: Lung disease (without specification).

Tetrachlorobenzodioxine:

C: Chloracne,

Tetrachloroethane:

A: Vomiting, abdominal pains, cyanosis, asphyxia, anorexia, conjunctivitis, fever, albuminuria, rhinitis, salivation, death.

C: Delirium, convulsions, haemolysis, heart disease, kidney disease, taste disorders, tremor, fatty degeneration of liver, anaemia, oedema, ascites, polyneuropathia.

Tetrachloroethylene: see Perchloroethylene.

Tetrachloroquinone:

A: Conjunctivitis.

Tetraethyl lead:

A: Insomnia, hyperreflexia, hypotension, hallucinations, convulsions, fatigue, tremor, muscular spasms (facial), hypothermia, acute mania, arrythmia, gastro-intestinal disturbances, mydriasis, salivation, coma, death.

C: Nail dystrophia.

Th: Skin contamination: Immediate washing with petrol.
In all cases of intoxication Ca-EDTA (sodium-calciumedetate) intravenously 15-20 mg/kg bodyweight.

Tetraethyl-thiuram-disulphide:

A: Alcohol intolerance, anorexia, nausea, vomiting.

Tetrafluorethylene:

A simple asphyxiant, see Argon.

Tetrahydrofurane:

A: Conjunctivitis, bronchitis.

Tetrahydronaphthalene (tetraline):

C: Urine discolouration.

2,2,4,4-Tetramethyl-1,3-cyclobutanediol:

A: Skin dystrophia.

Tetramethylenecyanide:

A: Gastro-intestinal disturbances.

C: Loss of weight.

Tetramethyl lead:

A: Heart arrythmia, delirium, gastro-intestinal disturbances, hypotension, tremor, mydriasis, hypothermia.

C: Nail dystrophia.

Tetramethyl silane:

C: Conjunctivitis, corncal oedema, kidney disease.

Tetramethylthiuramdisulphide:

A: Alcohol intolerance, Antabus effect, nausea, vomiting.

Tetramethylthiuram-monosulphide: see Tetramethylthiuram-disulphide.

Tetranitromethane:

A: Conjunctivitis, bronchitis, pulmonary oedema.

C: Methaemoglobinaemia, liver damage.

Tetranitromethylaniline:

C: Epistaxis.

Tetryl:

C: Skin pigmentation, conjunctivitis, asthma, anaemia, gastro-intestinal disturbances, epistaxis, nausea, vomiting, abdominal pains, rhinitis.

Thallium:

A: Nausea, vomiting, general oedema, abdominal pains, joint pains, convulsions, diarrhoea, kidney injury, albuminuria, eosinophilia, hyperaesthesia, paraesthesia, delirium, coma, death.

C: Myocarditis, fatigue, severe pains in the calves of legs, lymphocytosis, alopecia, discolouration of hair, retrobulbar neuritis, ataxia, lens opacities, anorexia, constipation, polyneuropathia, anhidrosis, nail dystrophia (Lunulastreifen).

Thiocyanates:

C: Anaemia, CNS-disorders, nausea, vomiting, vertigo, rhinitis.

Thionyl chlorides:

A: Conjunctivitis, keratitis, skin burns.

Thiourea:

C: Anaemia, leucopenia, thrombopenia.

Thiurams:

A: Alcohol intolerance.

Thomas' slag dust:

A: Bronchitis, dyspnoea, haemoptysis, laryngitis, pharyngitis, pneumonia, psychiatric disturbances, rhinitis, pulmonary oedema.

C: Bronchitis, emphysema.

Thorium:

C: Cataract, extrapyramidal symptoms, lung fibrosis.

Tin (inorganic compounds):

C: Lung fibrosis ("stannosis").

Tin (organic compounds):

A: Corrosive to skin, phototoxic, keratitis.

Th: Skin resorption very important. n-Heptane is said to be the most effective rinsing agent.

Titanium tetrachloride:

A: Skin dystrophia.

TNT: see Trinitrotoluene.

Tobacco dust:

C: Rhinitis.

o-Tolidine see Benzidine.

Toluene:

A: Mild fatigue, weakness, exhilaration, confusion, paraesthesia, nausea, vomiting, headache, ataxia, taste disorders, coma, keratitis (corneal burns).

C: Anaemia, restlessness, leukaemia, leucopenia, liver disease, sleep disturbances, fatigue, loss of weight.

Toluene diamines:

A: Dermatitis.

C: Fatty degeneration of liver, jaundice, anaemia, haemolysis.

2,4-Toluene-diisocyanate:

A: Conjunctivitis, rhinitis, bronchitis, sweating, asthma bronchiale.

C: Fatigue, lung fibrosis, asthma, cyanosis, emphysema, liver disease.

p-Toluene-sulphonyl chloride:

A: Skin dystrophia, fatigue, coma, conjunctivitis, convulsions, headache, nausea, vomiting.

C: Jaundice, paralysis, anorexia, loss of weight.

Toluidines:

A: Dyspnoea, headache, miction disturbances, fatigue.

Trauma (mechanical, eyes):

A: Cataract.

Trichlorobenzenes:

A: Alopecia, dermatitis.

1,1,1-Trichloroethane:

A: Heart arrythmia, headache, fatigue.

1,1,2-Trichloroethane:

A: Conjunctivitis, ataxia, headache, somnolence.

Trichloroethylene:

A: Vertigo, alcohol intolerance, Antabus effect, heart arrythmia, myopathia, somnolence, coma, conjunctivitis, skin flush (together with ethanol ingestion), headache.

C: Miction disturbances, skin dystrophia, psychiatric disturbances, polyneuropathia, papilloedema, neuralgia n. trigemini.

Trichloronitromethane:
A: Bronchitis, conjunctivitis, nausea, pulmonary oedema.
C: Sulphaemoglobinaemia.

Tri-o-cresyl-phosphate:
A: Abdominal pain, diarrhoea, pains of hands and feet.
C: Latency 1-3 weeks after acute exposure. Motor polyneuropathia (similar to poliomyelitis), ataxia, gastro-intestinal disturbances.

Triethylenemelamine:
C: Gastro-intestinal disturbances, leucopenia.

Triethylenetetramine:
A: Dermatitis.

Trifluorobromomethane:
A: Bronchitis.

Trifluorochloroethylene:
C: Kidney and liver disease.

Trimethylbenzenes:
A: Fatigue.
C: Thrombocytopenia, epistaxis, bronchospasm, headache, bronchitis.

Trimethylbismuthine:
C: Encephalopathia (similar to organic lead compounds).

Trimethylenetrinitramine:
A: coma, convulsions, insomnia, restlessness.
C: Convulsions.

Trinitromethane:
A: Headache, nausea, vomiting.

Trinitrotoluene:
C: Discolouration of hair, cyanosis, jaundice, met- and sulphaemoglobinaemia, gastro-intestinal disturbances, liver disease, papilloedema.

Trisodiumphosphate:
A: Skin dystrophia.

Tulips (bulbs and flowers):
C: Nail dystrophia.

Tungsten (Wolfram):
A: Bronchitis, cough, dyspnoea.
C: Lung fibrosis.

Turpentine:
A: Bronchitis, conjunctivitis, convulsions, cough, dyspnoea, vertigo, kidney injury.
C: Kidney injury.

Ultra sound:

A: Tinnitus, fatigue, vertigo, nausea, vomiting, psychiatric disturbances, somnolence.

Uranium:

C: Nephritis, hepatic degeneration.

Urethane: see Ethyl carbamate.

UV-light (Welding arcs, mercury vapour lamps):

A: Conjunctivitis, keratitis.

C: Skin pigmentation.

Vanadium:

A: Hypertension, somnolence, bronchospasm, dimness of vision, tremor, blindness, convulsions, diarrhoea, anaemia, anorexia, nausea, vomiting, emaciation, epistaxis, haemoptysis, conjunctivitis, bronchitis, coma.

C: Conjunctivitis, dyspnoea, greenish discolouration of the tongue, chest pain, nail dystrophia, tremor in fingers and arms, reticulation of lungs (X-ray), melancholia, keratitis, corneal oedema, dental discoloration.

Th: Symptomatic. BAL seems to be of some use. Vitamin C could be tried.

Vegetable dust:

C: Rhinitis, asthma.

Vibrating tools:

C: Decalcification of bones in carpus, injuries to soft tissues (Dupuytren's contracture), osteomalacia, Raynaud's phenomenon, pains of hands, sclerodermia.

Vinyl chloride (monomer):

A: Hyperaesthesia, headache, hyperhidrosis, dermographia, fatigue.

C: Anaemia, Raynaud's phenomenon, liver function disturbances, liver angiosarcoma, acroosteolysis, sclerodermia.

Vinyl ether:

C: Liver disease.

Vinyl pyridine:

A: Irritation of skin, bronchitis, conjunctivitis.

Vinyl toluene:

A: Conjunctivitis.

C: Kidney and liver damage.

Water:

A: Ingestion combined with NaCl depletion: Nausea, vomiting.

Th: Sodium chloride.

Water glass:

A: Skin dystrophia.

Welding (arc-):

A: Conjunctivitis.

C: Skin pigmentation.

White spirit:

A: Coma, conjunctivitis, convulsions, headache, nausea, vomiting, skin dystrophia.

Wood dust:

C: Asthma, conjunctivitis, rhinitis.

Xenon:

A simple asphyxiant, see Argon.

Xylenes:

A: Narcosis, fatigue, vertigo, inebriation, shivering, dyspnoea, nausea, vomiting, unconsciousness.

C: Rhinitis, liver disease, cardiovascular disorders, conjunctivitis, epistaxis, meno-metrorrhagia, anaemia, leucopenia, thrombocytopenia.

Xylidine:

A: "Blood disorders" (without specification).

C: Liver disease.

Zinc chloride:

A: Bronchitis, dermatoses, skin ulcers, perforation of nasal septum.

Zinc diethyl-dithiocarbamate:

A: Conjunctivitis, rhinitis, pharyngitis.

Zinc dimethyl-dithiocarbamate: see Zinc diethyl-dithio carbamate.

Zinc ethylene bis-(dithio carbamate):

A: Dermatitis.

Zinc oxide:

A: Dermatitis.

Zinc stearate:

A: Fever, shivering.

Zirconium:

C: Lung granulomata, lung fibrosis.

BIBLIOGRAPHY

Adams, R. M.: Occupational Contact Dermatitis, J. B. Lippincott & Co., Philadelphia & Toronto 1969.

Cahiers et Notes Documentaires, Institut National de Recherche et Securité, Paris 1969-1973.

Carlsson, A. & Hultengren, M.: Metabolism of ^{14}C-labelled Methylene Chloride in Rats, Stockholm 1974.

Deichman, W. B.: Health Hazards in Farming and Gardening, American Medical Association 1972.

Ebbehöj, J. & Reumert, T.: General Principles in Treatment of Chemical Injuries, Danish Environmental Protection Agency, Copenhagen 1975.

Encyclopedia of Occupational Health and Safety, I.L.O., Geneva 1971.

Fregert, S.: Manual of Contact Dermatitis, Munksgaard, Copenhagen 1974.

Hamilton, A. & Hardy, Harriet L.: Industrial Toxicology, Publishing Sciences Group Inc., U.S.A., 1974.

Holstein, E.: Grundriss der Arbeitsmedizin, Johan Ambrosius Verlag, Leipzig 1969.

Hunter, D.: The Diseases of Occupations, The English Universities Press, London 1975.

Jacobs, M. B.: The Analytical Chemistry of International Poisons, Hazards and Solvents, Interscience Publishers Inc., New York 1949.

Kinnersley, P.: The Hazards of Work, Pluto Press, London 1973.

Moeschlin, S.: Klinik und Therapie der Vergiftungen, Georg Thieme Verlag, Stuttgart 1972.

Notes on the Diagnosis of Occupational Diseases, HMSO London 1972.

Parkes, R.: Occupational Lung Disorders, Butterworth & Co., London 1974.

Patty, F. A.: Industrial Hygiene and Toxicology, vol. II, Interscience Publishers, New York 1967.

Sax, N. Irving: Dangerous Properties of Industrial Materials, Van Nostrand Reinhold Comp., New York 1975.

Shepard, T. H.: Catalog of Teratogenic Agents, The Johns Hopkins University Press, Baltimore and London 1973.

Trevethick, R. A.: Environmental and Industrial Health Hazards, William Medical Books Ltd., London 1973.

Zenz, Carl: Occupational Medicine, Year Book Medical Publishers, Chicago 1975.

Articles and Reviews from Journals of Occupational Hygiene, Health and Safety.

Personal communications.

The following agent was omitted from your book:

The following citation in the book is inaccurate:

The following citation should be added under the heading of:

References:

Authors:

Journal or book:

Vol.   page   year

Publisher of book:

Comments:

Signed

Address

Send to:

Dr. J. Daugaard

c/o Munksgaard Int. Publishers Ltd.
35, Nr. Søgade
DK-1370 Copenhagen K

DENMARK